THE PROSTATE CANCER ESSENTIALS FOR SURVIVAL SERIES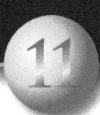

# LYMPH NODE POSITIVE PROSTATE CANCER

## MICHAEL J. DATTOLI, MD

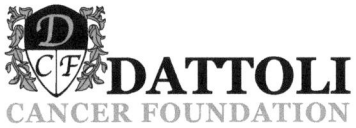

SARASOTA, FLORIDA

*Prostate Cancer Essentials for Survival Series: Lymph Node Positive Prostate Cancer*

Copyright © 2022–2025 by Michael J. Dattoli

All rights reserved. No part of this work may be reproduced or transmitted in any form or by any means, electronic or mechanical, including photocopying or recording, or by any information storage or retrieval system, except as may be expressly permitted by the 1976 Copyright Act or in writing by the publisher.

ISBN-10: 9-983741-66-3
ISBN-13: 978-1-9837-4166-1

Published by the Dattoli Cancer Foundation, Sarasota, FL

Book design and composition by Daniel van Loon, Batavia, IL
Book edits and revisions by Design Corps, Colorado Springs, CO

# MEDICAL DISCLAIMER

This book is intended as a supplement but not as a substitute for the medical advice of a physician. It is imperative that you consult a qualified healthcare professional with regard to all matters relating to your health and particular situation. Neither the publisher nor the authors bear responsibility for any consequences due to the reader's decision to use any particular treatment, medication, dietary supplement or other healthcare practices discussed in this book.

# DEDICATION

This booklet is dedicated to all those whose lives have been touched by prostate cancer, and to the patients and their families whom we are privileged to serve and educate as cancer care providers.

# ACKNOWLEDGMENTS

We are deeply grateful to a number of people who have contributed to this booklet in a number of ways. Our thanks to Greg Lawrence, for his editorial efforts and to Ginya Carnahan, Chris Wells, and Jone Fay at the Dattoli Cancer Center & Brachytherapy Research Institute for their ongoing assistance.

We deeply appreciate all of those wonderful patients and family members who have contacted the Dattoli Cancer Foundation for counseling and guidance and in turn have given us their support and encouragement. It is your spirit and commitment in confronting this disease that inspires us all.

# CONTENTS

**INTRODUCTION: Management of Lymph Node Positive Prostate Cancer** ............ 9
  *The Complementary Roles of Diagnostic Imaging and Advanced Radiotherapy* ............................... 9

**ONE: Diagnosing and Treating Positive Lymph Nodes** ................................................ 13

**TWO: Salvage Radiation versus Adjuvant Radiation Therapy** ...................................... 20
  *Historical Perspective Derived from Evidence-based Data* ....................................... 20

**THREE: Local and Regional Diagnostic Tools** ................................................. 28
  *Local Diagnostic Staging Studies* ................................................................. 28
  *Regional/Distant Diagnostic Staging Studies* ...................................................... 29
  *Combidex Results* ................................................................................. 29
  *Tracking the 4th Dimension* ....................................................................... 30

**FOUR: Updates on Current Feraheme USPIO Status and New MRI Contrast Agents for Lymph Node Imaging** ................................... 33

**FIVE: Raising the Radiation Dose** .............................................................. 36

**SIX: DART and Biologic-Directed Radiation** ..................................................... 38
  *DART and Tumor Dose Escalation/Urethral Dose Demodulation Using Fusion Techniques* ............ 38
  *Treating Abdominal or Para-aortic Nodes* ......................................................... 40

**SEVEN: Comparing Primary Treatment Options for High Risk Patients** ................. 41
  *Surgery versus Combination Protocol Radiotherapy* ............................................. 41

## APPENDICES ............ 45

*A: Independent Review and Summary of 16-year Data ............ 45*
*B: Dattoli Lymph Node Imaging Studies ............ 49*
*C: Dr. Dattoli on Treating Metastatic Disease ............ 53*
*D: Glossary of Medical Terms ............ 59*

*About the Author ............ 73*
*The Dattoli Cancer Foundation Mission ............ 74*
*Order More Booklets in the Series ............ 75*
*The Warning Signs of Prostate Cancer ............ 76*

# INTRODUCTION

# MANAGEMENT OF LYMPH NODE POSITIVE PROSTATE CANCER

## The Complementary Roles of Diagnostic Imaging and Advanced Radiotherapy

The poet Ralph Waldo Emerson once said, *"Build a better mousetrap and the world will beat a path to your door."* If the mouse is prostate cancer, we've been working on that trap for many years now and have made great progress diagnosing and treating this disease, even with cases where the cancer has spread outside the prostate gland.

The subject of this booklet is how recent innovations with diagnostic imaging techniques and radiation delivery technologies are enabling us to effectively treat men whose prostate cancer has invaded their lymph nodes—men who most physicians in this field previously thought were incurable and had limited treatment options. As we shall see, considerable progress is being made with these patients. While exploring the diagnosis and treatment of lymph node positive prostate cancer, we will also discuss prostate cancer treatment options that can help most newly diagnosed prostate cancer patients avoid lymph node disease.

We will show you how this can now be accomplished with state-of-the-art radiation therapy utilized as a primary treatment for those patients who are at risk for lymph node disease. Other booklets in this series, including *The Dattoli Prostate Cancer Challenge*, explore all the currently available treatment options for newly diagnosed patients and our own successful protocol of DART (Dynamic Adaptive Radiotherapy) combined with brachytherapy (radioactive seed implantation). This booklet includes a summary of our 16-year results treating intermediate and high-risk patients with our combination radiotherapy protocol.

Many of the advances of the past decade, perhaps most importantly the evolution of DART, have allowed thousands of men to be treated non-surgically with every expectation of surviving with high quality of life for many years, without experiencing a biological recurrence of the disease. We often remind our patients and their families that the newest life expectancy tables are very encouraging: a man who is 65 years old today is predicted to live an average of 18 more years, if he is 70 that prediction is more than 14 years, and if he is 75 he is expected to live more than 11 years. We want to ensure that a diagnosis of prostate cancer will not have an impact on men living out their lives to the full as expected.

Men who have chosen a treatment other than our combination radiation protocol to treat their prostate cancer, especially those having a robotic surgical procedure, often face a different future. In our practice, we are seeing alarming numbers of post-robotic patients coming to us for salvage radiation as soon as 6 to 10 months after having surgery. In addition to postsurgical patients, we are also seeing men treated elsewhere who experience recurrence after cryosurgery, high intensity frequency ultrasound (HIFU), and radiation, both full course external radiation and brachytherapy. Recurrence, or more precisely, "persistence" of disease, is obvious when the PSA fails to fall after surgery, or if it falls but soon begins to rise again. In these cases, prostate cancer had probably already spread outside the prostate, and therefore the robotic procedure was not successful in removing all the active cancer cells. When cancer is left behind after surgery, there is also a significant risk that the lymph nodes will be involved.

Among some of our own patients who were treated more than a decade ago, even though their PSA reached an appropriate nadir value less than 0.2, a small percentage of men are seeing a slow rise of PSA many years after their initial treatment, indicating that some few cells must have escaped the original course of radiation therapy. We addressed this potentiality more than a decade ago by adding a third phase to our tailored combination treatment. This third phase involves directing additional radiation to the periprostatic tissue as well as to relevant lymph nodes, as they are the usual routes of escape for cancer cells. In this way, we make sure that we are treating those areas where cancer is most likely to have spread outside the gland.

Fortunately, advances with diagnostic imaging have kept pace with our treatment capabilities utilizing the most sophisticated forms of radiation therapy. Working with leading radiologists, we now employ a number of contrast agents and fusion techniques for enhanced imaging. These are used in conjunction with MRI and CT scans, as well as with positron emission tomography (PET) scans. One bright star among others in this realm is the USPIO (Ultra-Small Super-Paramagnetic Iron Oxide) imaging test. This test involves an intravenous infusion of radioactive nanoparticles such as Ferumoxytal (Feraheme), which makes it possible for us to obtain a very revealing picture of exactly where active prostate cancer cells have traveled through the lymph system.

Over the past decade, we blazed a trail for lymphatic node identification and subsequent radiation treatment in partnership with radiologist Dr. Stephen Bravo and his colleagues formerly at Sand Lake Imaging in Orlando, Florida. We are steadily gathering and publishing data in the hope of future FDA approval of the USPIO test, paving the way for wider availability among physicians and increased insurance reimbursement (see our published results below). The process of obtaining FDA approval can be long and tedious, but we are steadily working toward that goal.

In a recent presentation at a symposium sponsored by the American Society of Therapeutic Radiation Oncology (ASTRO), we reported on our encouraging progress. In summary, 33 of 36 patients with biochemical recurrence of prostate cancer (evidenced by rising PSA) were identified with positive lymph nodes through the USPIO testing process, and those positive nodes were verified by subsequent biopsy, validating the accuracy of the test. The USPIO technology has the ability to identify positive nodes down to a resolution of 3-4 mm, and in some cases even to 1-2 mm.

These imaging tests help us detect possible sites of recurrent prostate cancer that more conventional tests can't identify. Locating recurrent prostate cancer allows us to identify small, isolated deposits of cancer—both within and outside the prostate—that can be targeted for more effective treatment. This is indeed good news for those men who after treatment experience an otherwise unexplained rise in PSA that suggests recurrent cancer.

A recent study from the University of Pennsylvania confirmed our published findings and reported that ongoing clinical trials utilizing Feraheme as an MRI contract agent are promising (Repurposing Ferumoxytol: Diagnostic and therapeutic applications of an FDA-approved nanoparticle, Theranostics 2022; 12(2):796-816). These researchers observed, "Moreover, ferumoxytol holds great promise for many other biomedical applications including MRI, drug delivery, oral biofilm treatment, and anti-cancer and anti-inflammatory therapies."

These state-of-the-art imaging techniques can identify lymph node spread in patients initially treated for high-risk disease, and they are already allowing us to effectively treat patients with positive lymph nodes by utilizing DART. Our expectation is to further increase our cure rate in this group of patients by treating lymph nodes which may otherwise have not been detected and located with specificity without the benefit of the USPIO/MRI scanning and/or contrast-enhanced MRI and CT imaging.

These diagnostic advances have tremendous potential for improving overall survival of recurrent prostate cancer patients, and also for identifying and treating otherwise undetected cancer in pelvic and abdominal lymph nodes of patients presenting at first diagnosis with high-risk, aggressive prostate cancer. Such breakthroughs are helping us to determine which cancers are tigers and which are pussycats—which are highly aggressive and which are more contained and more easily treated.

What we are finding is that we can control lymph node disease better with this approach to treatment. In many ways, control can be as effective as cure. We don't cure diabetes or hypertension or a host of other diseases, but we can control them. So if we can control prostate cancer with these patients who have regionally-advanced disease, we believe they will benefit both in terms of survival and quality of life.

## Research studies that have reported our findings to date with USPIO include the following:

Yun Rose Li, Michael J. Dattoli, Jelle Barentsz, Mack Roach III, *Radiotherapy guided by ultra small superparamagnetic iron oxide (USPIO)-contrast MRI staging for patients with advanced or recurrent prostate cancer*, submitted to the American Society of Clinical Oncology (ASCO) for featured conference presentations in February, 2020 (see Appendix B of this booklet).

Dattoli MJ, Bravo SM, Kaplon DM, Hayes M, Osorio A, Dycus PM, Bostwick D, Kaminski JM, *Efficacy of Feraheme as Lymphatic Contrast Agent in Prostate Cancer*; featured presentations at the February 2018 annual symposiums of the American Society of Clinical Oncology (ASCO) and the Annual Symposium on Clinical Interventional Oncology (CIO) (see Appendix B of this booklet).

Bravo, S.M., Dattoli, M.J., Myers, C.E., et al; *Safety and Efficacy of Feraheme as a Lympatic Contrast Agent*. ASTRO Symposia. Atlanta, GA, October 2013.

Bravo, S.M., Dattoli, M.J., Myers, C.E., et al; *Ferumoxytol as a Lymph Node Contrast Agent in Patients with Metastatic Prostate Carcinoma: Rad-Path Correlation, including presentation*. ASTRO Symposia. Orlando, FL, February 2013.

Bravo, S.M., Dattoli, M.J. Myers, C.E., et al: *Ferumoxytol as a Lymph Node Contrast Agent in Patients with Metastatic Prostate Carcinoma: Rad-Path Correlation, including presentation*, Radiologic Sciences of North America, Chicago, Illinois, Novermber 2012

Bravo, S.M., Dattoli, M.J., Myers, C.E., et al; *Potential for Feraheme as Lymphatic Contrast Imagine Agent*. Submitted to RSNA November 2011.

Bravo, S.M., Dattoli, M.J., Myers, C.E., et al; *Safety of Ferumoxytol (Feraheme) in Patients with Prostate Carcinoma*. Submitted to RSNA November 2011.

Bravo, S.M., Dattoli, M.J., Myers, C.E., et al; *Ferumoxytol as Lymph Node Contrast Agent in Patients with Metastic Prostate Carcinoma: Rad-Path Correlation*. Submitted to RSNA November 2011.

# CHAPTER ONE

# DIAGNOSING AND TREATING POSITIVE LYMPH NODES

The approach taken by most other physicians when prostate cancer invades the lymph system is not curative. They usually subscribe to the belief that when cancer has spread to the lymph nodes, it is incurable. But why should prostate cancer in the lymph nodes be approached any differently than breast cancer in the lymph nodes, cervical cancer in the lymph nodes or the other common cancers that often spread to the lymph nodes? All of the cancers listed in the box below lend themselves to a curative approach by physicians, and we have come to believe that positive lymph nodes with prostate cancer should also be treated with curative intent.

### Other malignancies commonly associated with lymph nodes
Breast Cancer + lymph nodes → treat with curative intent
Colorectal Cancer + lymph nodes → treat with curative intent
Head & Neck Cancers + lymph nodes → treat with curative intent
Hodgkin's Lymphoma → treat with curative intent
Bronchogenic Cancer + lymph nodes → treat with curative intent
**Prostate Cancer + lymph nodes → Incurable?** *We don't think so!*

Granted, until recently there was no truly effective way, other than by biopsy, to identify the specific nodes that harbor active prostate cancer. With literally dozens of lymph nodes upstream from the prostate gland, individual biopsies, sampling or especially surgical removal (dissection) of each suspect gland, could result in significant morbidity (lower extremity and pelvic lymphodema). In the best circumstances, some oncologists and urologists would try to identify the abdominal nodes using CT scans and Prostascint®; both of these tests are associated with a high rate of false positive results, especially when lymph nodes are 1.0 cm or smaller. Usually only those nodes closest to the prostate gland are determined to be positive. In our practice, the Prostascint® test has for the most part been replaced by other advanced techniques, such as USPIO, C-11 Choline PET/CT, C-11 Carbon Acetate PET/CT, and more recently, MRI scans utilizing UniMark and/or UniRay contrast agents. We favor the USPIO test and other contrast-enhanced MRI scans because most of the others have been fraught with false positive results.

The lymph system that can be invaded by prostate cancer is quite extensive. A large radiation oncology group defined standards of care for prostate cancer (Lawson et al, Int. J. Rad Onc, 74(2) 383-387, 2009). They listed the following pelvic lymph nodes as being at high risk for developing cancer:

- Distal common iliacs
- Pre-sacral
- External iliacs
- Internal iliacs
- Obturator

As pictured below, the nodes basically follow the vascular pattern of blood circulation from the para-aortic region and down. That's the lay of the land, so to speak, where prostate cancer spreads, the area that involves the lymph nodes.

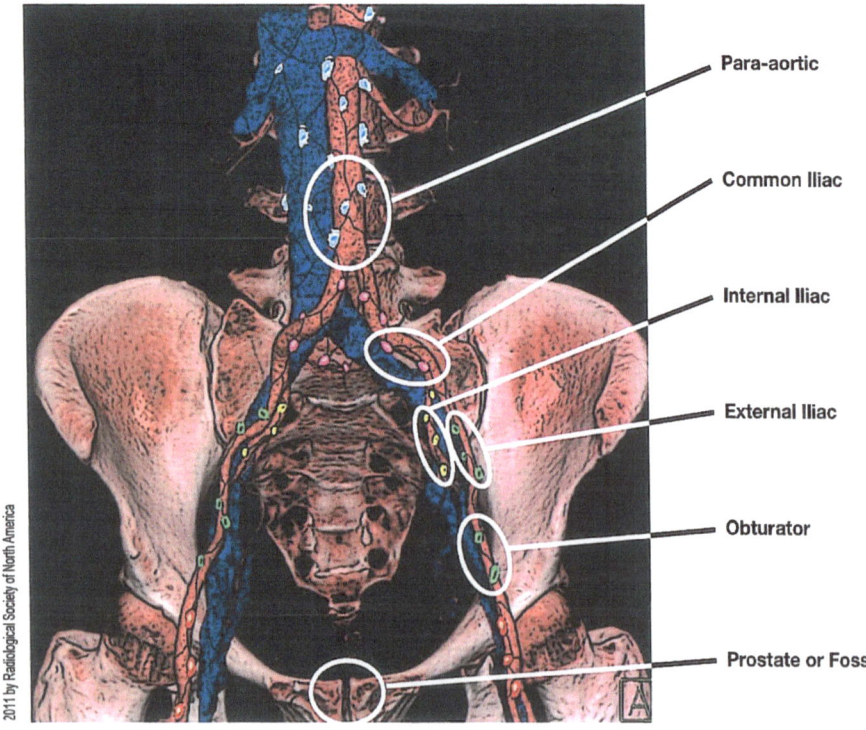

Paño B et al. Radiographics 2011;31:135-160    RadioGraphics

If you are diagnosed with positive lymph node prostate cancer, you may be put on hormonal therapy and told to put your affairs in order. If lymph node positive disease is identified, those patients have historically been treated with hormonal therapies, systemic chemotherapy and various clinical trials in the hope of stopping or slowing the advance of active cells through the lymph system. (Chemotherapy was a last-ditch effort prior to the availability of a new breed of last-resort drugs such as Zytiga® and Xtandi®).

Two advances in diagnosis and treatment of prostate cancer were occurring simultaneously in the past decade that now make accurate identification and targeted radiation to those nodes possible and practical. In terms of diagnosis, almost as a fluke, a previously FDA-approved treatment for unrelated chronic kidney disease demonstrated the ability to highlight lymph nodes containing active prostate cancer cells; not just the nodes in close proximity to the prostate gland (pelvic region), but those higher in the abdomen, such as the para aortic and aorta caval, and even those lymph nodes in the mediastinum (chest region) and neck. This is the USPIO test utilizing Feraheme. We anticipate continuing clinical trails in the future with Feraheme.

This diagnostic breakthrough uses a molecule (nanoparticle) called Ferumoxytol, more commonly referred to as Feraheme, which is infused to identify the affected lymph nodes with a high degree of accuracy (95% or higher). Thus, there is no need for morbid lymph node biopsies, sampling or dissection.

The location of these affected lymph nodes, above the diaphragm and up as high as the clavicle, had previously proven to be out of the range for traditional broad spectrum radiation. Constant movement in the chest and the location of specific sensitive organs (kidneys, liver, lungs, heart) would pose virtually impossible obstacles to effective radiation treatment at the necessary higher dose levels required to eradicate the cancer. And morbidity would have been overwhelming with earlier radiation delivery technologies.

However, with the advent of DART radiation dynamically adjusting the microbeams to organ motion in real time (specialized radiotherapy created by and available only at the Dattoli Cancer Center), these lymph nodes can now be successfully irradiated to halt the advance of prostate cancer through the lymph system, without exposing the critical organs to any damaging radiation exposure. Treatment of lymph nodes above the diaphragm may be extremely effective in ameliorating symptoms associated with castrate-resistant prostate cancer, and even afford some patients extended biochemical disease-free survival.

We only have to look at the survival statistics for lymph node positive patients with other cancers to predict the potential success of this approach with prostate cancer patients. Prostate cancer generally affects areas near the center of the body, with the prostate located in close proximity to the bladder and the rectum, but so does cervical cancer. A study published in 1995 cited 10-year survival results for patients with lymph node positive cervical cancer. Without any lymph node radiation, only 50% of these patients survived even 5 years. However, there was 55% survival at 10 years when pelvic and para-aortic nodes were irradiated, and 44% survival at 10 years when just the pelvic nodes were irradiated (RTOG 7920, JAMA, 274 (5): 387-93, 1995). Those results are summarized as follows:

### RTOG 7920 Ten Year Treatment Results
➤ Overall Survival 55%—pelvic + para-aortic lymph nodes
➤ Overall Survival 44%—pelvic lymph nodes only

*That 11% difference in survival at ten years is statistically significant.*

Studies like the RTOG study on cervical cancer cited above are termed "evidence-based data." What that means is we take two patients who have similar disease and one patient goes behind Door Number One to have one type of treatment (typically the "standard treatment"), and the other patient goes behind Door Number Two to have a different type of treatment, and they both come back in five to ten years and we see how they are. The significance of those results can't be denied. And this is what we follow in medicine and this is how our knowledge of therapies grows over the years. We look at these studies and often ask how we can do better than these evidence-based trials.

Let's turn our attention again to prostate cancer. We expect similar or greater benefit for prostate cancer patients as that cervical cancer study reported, since the location of the nodes was unknown as compared to the USPIO-defined nodes (which can be boosted with DART to receive an even higher dose level of radiation). We will publish additional results as soon as our data has matured to the point where we have a statistically significant number of patients in our study with a substantive median follow-up. Who would benefit most from nodal radiation treatment? Patients who have lymph node involvement after surgery and other patients who have high risk factors would stand to benefit from nodal radiation, as indicated below:

## Those Benefited by Nodal Radiation

➤ **Post-surgical patients having adverse features**
  • Clinical Stage T3 disease (especially seminal vesicle involvement and also patients having positive surgical margins)
  • High Gleason Score (especially 8-10)
  • pN1 disease (patients diagnosed with positive lymph nodes)

➤ **High-Risk, Intact Prostate Cancer**
  • Clinical Stage T3 disease (especially seminal vesicle involvement)
  • PSA $\geq$ 20 ng/ml
  • Gleason Score 8-10)

The following evidence-based trials got us to where we are today with treating lymph nodes. The first was RTOG 7506, which was led by Dr. Gerald Hanks at the Fox Chase Cancer Center. He thought outside the box, so to speak. He suggested treating the para-aortic lymph nodes for patients having N1 disease (positive pelvic lymph nodes) with external radiation. This is known as extended field radiation. Patients were not given Androgen Deprivation Therapy (ADT) and the radiation therapy predated 3D Conformal Radiation (3DCRT). Dr. Hanks and his team found that after 5 years 63% of patients were surviving and almost 30% at ten years.

## Supportive Data for Extended Field Radiation
## for intact locally advanced nodal disease

**RTOG 7506** (randomized 90 patients)
  Phase III Study for T3 N1 disease
    Arm 1   Pelvic radiation only
    Arm 2   Pelvic + para-aortic radiation
    Overall survival at 5 years = 63%  (vs. 27% Arm 1)
    Overall survival at 10 years = 29%  (vs. 7% Arm 1)
    60Gy Median Dose

*Hanks et al, Int J Rad Onc, 40 (4) 765-8, 1998*

A similar study was conducted at the Memorial Sloan-Kettering Cancer Center that reported similar results treating N1 disease with extended nodal radiation. At 15 years, they reported 34% overall survival and 45% local control (*Lee et al, Urol 43: 640-644, 1994, MSKCC*). Those two studies exceeded expectations and flew in the face of conventional wisdom at the time. They opened the door to the path we are currently following by treating lymph nodes.

Back in 1995, Dr. Samuel Hellman at the Harvard Medical School did a multi-organ study on various cancers that had spread to other parts of the body such as the liver and lungs. He found that removing the cancer burden from those distant sites had a statistically significant impact on disease-free survival (Hellman et al, J Clin. Onc, 12: 8, 1995).

During the next decade, Dr. Deepinder Singh and his team at the University of Rochester Medical Center looked specifically at prostate cancer that had spread to the bones, and they found that patients who had 5 or fewer bone lesions could not only be treated but cured. That caused quite a stir in the field. Now patients with 5 lesions treated with radiation weren't necessarily cured, but the treatment did improve control of the cancer. Some patients with only 1 to 2 bones lesions were actually cured, and that was unheard of at the time (Singh et al, Int J. Rad Onc, 58: 3, 2004)

That finding opened the way for a number of clinical trials that involve identifying and treating patients with 5 or fewer metastatic lesions, which is called oligometastatic disease:

## Recent and Ongoing Clinical Trials
**Patients with Oligometastatic Disease at Presentation**
- ClinicalTrials.gov NCTO1345539, U. Pittsburgh, opened June 2011
- Non-systemic Treatment for Patients with Low Volume Metastatic Cancer
- ClinicalTrials.gov NCTO1558427, U. Hospital Ghent, Belgium, opened Feb. 2013
- Radiotherapy for Oligometastatic Prostate Cancer, ClinicalTrials.gove, NCTO1859221, U. Florida, Opened May 2013

Who will benefit the most from the advanced technologies we are currently using? The answer is patients having high-risk disease, and also postsurgical patients having adverse features, such as Gleason 8–10 and/or rising PSA's, which may also include seminal vesicle or lymph nodes invasion. With DART enhanced by advanced imaging techniques, we are already treating patients with oligometastatic disease affecting the bones (patients with 5 or fewer bony lesions) and the lungs (patients with 1 or 2 lung metastases). These state-of the-art technologies will also benefit patients for whom external radiation or brachytherapy have failed. Many of these patients can be treated with salvage Dynamic Adaptive Radiation Therapy

(DART). The disease in these cases may not be so advanced, and these patients may have a second chance for a cure.

The illustration below shows how with oligometastatic patients after surgery, we can treat the prostate bed where the gland was removed and enlarge the radiation target area to include the pelvic lymph nodes. As illustrated by the two images on the left side of the box, with advanced imaging that utilizes nanoparticle technology (which we will discuss in greater detail), we can pinpoint with a high degree of accuracy exactly which lymph nodes have been invaded by cancer. By increasing the size of the treatment box as illustrated by the four images on the right side of the box, we can treat more of the lymph nodes.

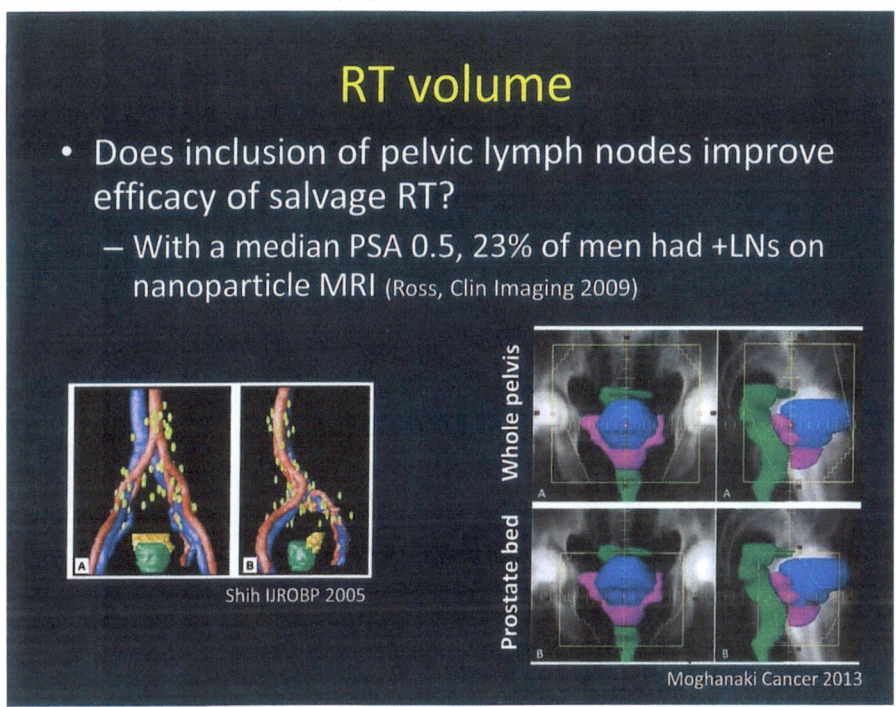

This is important for postsurgical patients whose PSA rises to 0.5 because 23% of those men had positive lymph node disease as revealed by nanoparticle MRI (magnetic resonance imaging) studies. All of those men stand to benefit from the use of nanoparticles and other contrast agents to locate affected lymph nodes, which can then be treated effectively with DART.

# CHAPTER TWO

# SALVAGE RADIATION VERSUS ADJUVANT RADIATION THERAPY

## Historical Perspective Derived from Evidence-based Data

After surgery, if the PSA rises to a certain point, patients may be treated with radiation and/or hormonal therapy. In that case, the radiation is a salvage therapy (SRT), which attempts to cure patients after surgery has failed. Adjuvant radiation therapy (ART) is planned in advance for surgical patients identified to have adverse features within the postoperative pathological specimens. It is planned that these patients will receive post-operative radiation 8 to 12 weeks after they have surgery. Surveys show that less than 15% of urologists refer patients for adjuvant radiation and/or hormonal therapy, so those options are underutilized.

Here we will summarize the results of a number of studies that investigated adjuvant and salvage radiation therapy, as well as hormonal therapy. One National Cancer Institute (NCI) trial reported that after surgery when the PSA reached 0.21 to 0.5, 48% of patients who received salvage radiation survived at 6 years. The percentage of patients surviving fell to only 8% when the PSA rose to 1.51. So the earlier patients are treated after the PSA begins to rise post-surgery the better the outcome with salvage radiation. What the study shows, summarized below, is how even that incremental rise in PSA impacts the biochemical freedom of progression of disease and overall survival after salvage radiation.

### NCI Prostate Cancer SPORE Study
**Predicting Outcomes of Salvage Radiation**
Multi-institutional, 1,540 consecutive pT3 patients
➢ Endpoint PSA >0.2 ng/ml Following RP
**Results at 6 years**
  Overall 6 year biochemical free progression = 32%

48% when post-op PSA: 0.21–0.5
40% when post-op PSA: 0.51–1.0
28% when post-op PSA: 1.01–1.5
18% when post-op PSA: > 1.51
➤ Side effects: acute RTOG 3-4 toxicity and late Grade 3 < 4%
➤ Shortcoming: low RT dose, 70 Gy

**Conclusion:** Benefit of Salvage Radiation Inversely Correlated to PSA Level

*Stephenson et al, J Clin Onc, 25, 2055-61, 2007*

Another study (SWOG 87-94) published in 2009 compared patients who were given adjuvant radiation 8 to 12 months after surgery with patients who received salvage radiation and hormones later after their PSA began to rise following surgery. These researchers reported that at 12.7 years follow-up, the patients who received adjuvant radiation had a 59% survival rate, while patients who received salvage radiation therapy had a 48% survival rate. That shows that adjuvant radiation really has a statistically significant impact, as summarized below.

Between the two groups of patients there was no statistical difference with side effects involving urination, bowels and erectile function. This finding is consistent with numerous other past and ongoing studies. In other words, a man's quality of life after having surgery will not be altered by subsequent radiation therapy. Quality of life is not affected by postsurgical adjuvant or salvage radiation.

## Supportive Data for Postsurgical Adjuvant Radiation Therapy (ART)

**SWOG 87-94:** (Randomized Clinical Trial – Long Term Follow-up)
➤ Adjuvant radiation therapy for high-risk post-surgical prostate cancer
➤ Endpoint overall survival and metastasis-free survival
   425 consecutive patients
   Median follow-up 12.7 years

|  | MEDIAN OVERALL SURVIVAL | METASTASIS-FREE SURVIVAL |
|---|---|---|
| 214 patients (adjuvant RT, 60-64Gy) | 59% | 93/214 |
| 211 patients (observation – salvage RT upon failure + ADT) | 48% $p = 0.023$ | 114/211 $p = 0.034$ |

**Quality of Life:** No statistical difference between the two groups with urination/bowels/erectile function

**NOTE:** Doses 60-64Gy to "pelvic fossa," low by contemporary standards.

*Thompson et al, J Urology: Vol 181, 956-62, 2009*

With this next study published in 2012, researchers followed one group of postsurgical patients who received radiation after their PSA rose to 0.2, and another group of postsurgical patients who were given radiation post-operatively (adjuvant). The results at 10 years were 61.% biochemical progression-free survival for the patients who received post-operative radiation versus 39.4% of patients who watched and waited until their PSA was rising before being treated with radiation. The 0.001 p value indicates the difference in outcomes was statistically significant.

---

**Supportive data for Adjuvant Radiation Therapy (ART)**

**EORTC 22911:**

Randomized 1,005 consecutive patients with pT3 disease, following RP
    Arm A—"Wait and see": (initiate post-op RT when PSA > 0.2)
    Arm B—adjuvant post-op RT (8 weeks median 64Gy, pre-3D-IMRT era)
    Median follow-up 10.6 years.

**Results**

10 year biochemical progression-free survival:
    Arm A—39.4%
    Arm B—61.8%
    $p = < 0.001$

**Arm B:** Also improved clinical progression-free survival; ($p = 0.009$), reduced local-regional failure ($p = 0.005$).

*Overall survival did not reach statistical significance ($p = 0.04$)*

**NOTE:** Nearly 50% of relapsing patients in the observation group received deferred radiation, yet the Arm B group will have had an advantage with biochemical disease free survival (the overall survival would likely have reached significance had this study continued).

Grade III toxicity 4.2% vs 2.6% ($p = 0.052$) Arm B

*Bolla et al, Lancet 380: 2018-27, 2012*

---

Another important study was conducted in Milan, Italy, and it tested adjuvant radiation combined with hormonal therapy versus hormonal therapy alone for postsurgical patients. The combined treatments of radiation and hormones are called a multi-modal approach. This trial was really asking the question does radiation have an impact.

95% and 86% of patients who received the radiation and hormones survived at 5 and 10 years respectively while 88% and 70% of patients who received hormones alone survived at 5 and 10 years respectively. Now these were patients who had positive lymph nodes after surgery, and again, the outcomes are statistically significant at 10 years, with a 16% difference for patients who had the radiation and hormones having better cancer specific survival.

## Milan Matched Analysis Trial

**Supportive data for both Post-op Radiation Therapy and ADT (multi-modal)**
Combination of Adjuvant Hormonal Therapy and Post-op Radiation Therapy prolongs survival in patients having pT2-4 pN1 prostate cancer:

**Results of matched analysis**
367 consecutive patients
  Group I—117 pT2-4  pN1 → ADT + RT (3DCRT)
  Group II—247 pT2-4  pN1 → ADT alone
Median follow-up 100.8 months

**Cancer Specific Survival**

|  | 5 YEARS | 10 YEARS |
|---|---|---|
| Group I (post-op ADT + RT) | 95% | 86% |
| Group II (post-op ADT alone) | 88% | 70% |
|  | $p = < 0.004$ |  |

*Briganti et al, European Urol, 59: 832-40, 2011) (Milan)*

The M.D. Anderson RTOG 85-31 study published in 2005 and summarized below followed patients with lymph node disease who either had a radical prostatectomy (RP) or their prostates were intact upon presentation. They were treated with a multi-modal approach. With two groups of patients, 488 received Adjuvant Radiation Therapy (RT) and hormones while 489 received radiation and hormones only after their PSA rose above 0.2. The first group fared better with surgery, radiation and hormones in terms of absolute survival, disease free survival, biochemical disease free survival, and even with patients having Gleason 7 to 10 scores.

## RTOG 85-31

Clinical stage pT3  pN1 disease treated with RT or RP + adjuvant vs delayed. In the RTOG 85-31 trial, patients received, neo-adjuvant 2 month ADT + during RT for bulky tumors resulting in statistical improvement in all end points (including Absolute Survival though only in Gleason scores $\leq 6$)
  977 randomized patients
  Arm I  488 patients – adjuvant ADT (begin final week of RT, then indefinitely)
  if RT—pelvic RT, 44-50Gy and 20-25Gy prostate boost

if RP—prostate bed treated to 60-65Gy

Arm II 489 patients—observation following RP/RT, ADT when loco-regional progression/distant mets or PSA ≥ 1.5

**Results:** Kaplan-Meier + Multivariate Cox Proportional hazard regression
Patients in Arm I benefited at 10 years vs Arm II
Absolute survival—48% vs 36% ($p < 0.03$)
Disease free survival—38% vs 23% ($p = 0.014$)
Biochemical disease survival—31% vs 9% ($p < 0.0001$)
**Gleason 7-10 survival—40% vs 30% ($p = 0.0039$)**

*Pilepich et al, Int J Rad Onc, Vol 61, No 5, 1285-90, 2005*

We are cautious about using hormonal therapy at our center because hormones do have some downsides with significant side effects, but this study and others have demonstrated that hormones can have significant advantages when combined with radiation.

Another study from the Fox Chase Cancer Center followed high-risk patients with Gleason scores 8-10 treated by pelvic radiation and hormonal therapy before and during radiation therapy, or by pelvic radiation combined with hormonal therapy (LH-RH) that continued 2 years after treatment. That study showed the patients who received post-radiation hormones for 2 years had an 81% survival rate versus 70% for those patients whose hormonal therapy ended immediately after radiation therapy (*Hanks et al, J Clin Onc, 21, 3972-8, 2003*). As noted, we are not overly enthusiastic about hormones, especially in the long term, but with the preponderance of data from various studies, we are obligated to offer hormonal therapy to patients, explaining the possible benefits and risks they can expect with hormones.

It should be noted that RTOG 92-02 reported similar survival rates with Gleason 8-10 patients, while the EORTC 22911 study showed that all Gleason scores benefited with respect to all endpoints except Overall Survival. The study showed prolonged biochemical disease-free survival and cancer specific survival. Gleason scores 8-10 appeared to benefit most.

Another evidence-based study, RTOG 96-01, showed the advantage of two years of hormonal therapy after surgery using 150 mg of Casodex. 57% of patients who received hormones showed no biochemical progression versus 40% who received a placebo instead of hormonal therapy. These two groups, of patients, arms 1 and 2, were followed a median of 7.1 years. Patients with Gleason scores 8 to 10 benefited the most. Some patients did have problems with gynecomastia, breast enlargement due to the Casodex. We do have various ways to deal with the gynecomastia problem. The researchers suggested a follow up study using a lower dose of that hormonal agent to 50 mg to see if that would alter the results. A related question now being studied is if the use of hormones can be reduced if the radiation dose is increased.

## RTOG 96-01

Randomized, multi-center trial comparing post-op salvage RT and 150mg Casodex for 2 years to post-op salvage RT and placebo in men with pT$_{2-3}$ N1 prostate cancer who have an elevated PSA after RP.

**Preliminary results:** (12/13/10)
  Median follow-up 7.1 years with 771 eligible patients
  Freedom from biochemical progression
  Arm 1—57% in EBRT + Casodex
  Arm 2—40% in EBRT + Placebo
  $p = < 0.003$

**Benefits greatest with Gleason 8-10 patients:** Gynecomastia problematic in the Casodex Arm 1 group. Question: would 50 mg Casodex demonstrate same impact?

*Ambrowitz et al, Semin Rad Onc 18: 15-22, 2008*

Finally, the EORTC 22863 study looked at patients with intact prostates, those who had not had surgery but had high risk features, such as Gleason scores 8 to 10. One group of patients was treated with pelvic radiation and given hormonal therapy in the form of an LH-RH agonist, while a second group of patients received pelvic radiation alone. They did find a statistically significant benefit with hormones. As you can see in the summary below, those who received hormonal therapy fared better in terms of 10-year overall survival and cancer specific survival than those patients who were not given hormones. We would be reluctant to use hormones for three years because of the risk of side effects problems. We would instead use a far more abbreviated hormonal regime (6 to 13 months). Hormones can exacerbate cardiovascular problems. Interestingly, this study found no cardiac incidents over a follow up period of 10 years.

So it appears there is a benefit using radiation (with or without hormones) with lymph node positive patients, but what about side effects? No trial using adjuvant radiation therapy (ART) and/or salvage radiation therapy (SRT) has demonstrated a statistically significant detriment to erectile function compared to radical prostatectomy alone. Nor has any ART or SRT trial demonstrated statistically significant bowel or bladder dysfunction without resolution at 2 to 5 years compared to baseline scores. *In fact, both ART and SRT trials are associated with < 1% radiation-related morbidities.* So the risk of side effects is remarkably low with radiation, not impacting what would otherwise be expected (quite contrary to what patients are often told).

## EORTC 22863

**High-Risk, Intact Locally Advanced Prostate Cancer**
**Stage T$_3$/T$_4$ or high-grade Gleason 8-10**
**415 consecutive patients randomized**
   **Group A—Pelvic RT alone (208)**
   **Group B—Pelvic RT + LH-RH agonist for 3 years (207)**

Median follow-up 10 years

|  | GROUP A |  | GROUP B |
|---|---|---|---|
| 10 year overall survival | 47% | vs | 39.8% (p = 0.0004) |
| Cancer specific survival | 30.4% | vs | 10.3% |

***No significant adverse cardiac events.***

Bolla et al, Lancet Oncol: 11: 1066-1073, 2010

And yet, even with the results of these major trials showing the benefits of radiation for surgery patients, only about 10% of urologists send their surgical patients for radiation. This is especially distressing when we consider the growing body of evidence supporting early postsurgical intervention with radiation.

Most studies suggest that salvage patients after surgery have approximately ten times the disease burden compared to patients treated with adjuvant radiation, and multiple prospective randomized trials have demonstrated a benefit for Adjuvant Radiation over Salvage Radiation. These comparison studies looked at Salvage Radiation with low PSA and especially Gleason scores 8 to10, seminal vesicle involvement, and positive margins (RTOG 7506; 8531, SWOG 8794; EORTC 29111). The multi-modal approach appears superior, increasing overall survival (RTOG 9202, RTOG 9601, EORTC 22863).

Salvage Radiation appears to be appropriate for patients who have the highest chance of having local regional disease:

- ➢ PSA doubling time > 12 months
- ➢ Positive surgical margins
- ➢ Interval to PSA failure ≥ 3 years
- ➢ Gleason 7 or lower

**So the take-home message for patients who have had surgery is don't wait too long to begin Salvage Radiation.** As a patient, you should be proactive with your urologist or oncologist, because many of them don't pay attention to the fact that if your PSA rises above 2.0, you're very unlikely to benefit from radiation or hormonal therapy or anything else. That number has been whittled down over the years, so it's now really between 0.2 and 0.6–after that, the results fall off for patients having successful outcomes.

Various studies are underway, but preliminary data suggests significant benefit to Adjuvant RT while the benefit of Salvage RT is inversely correlated to serum PSA at the time of RT. Patients with PSA values higher than 0.4 are less likely to be cured by Salvage RT. While there is still some uncertainty about Adjuvant versus Salvage radiation after surgery, the data shows that salvage is viable for most patients, but they have to keep a very close eye on the PSA to catch it rising early enough to get better results. That's very important to understand because it really is a matter of survival.

Doctors who see the rising PSA after surgery will often just monitor their patients with active surveillance, but that concept really shouldn't apply to postsurgical patients. It applies to newly diagnosed patients who have very low risk cancer, not to high-risk postsurgical patients. In any case, active surveillance doesn't mean just having your PSA checked once a year; it actually means biannually if not quarterly, as well as being biopsied at least once a year and having the PCA3 urine test. It also means undergoing periodical (annual or biannual) advanced imaging studies including but not limited to Multi-parametric MRIs and 3D Color-Flow Power Doppler Ultrasound, which we use at the Dattoli Cancer Center.

CHAPTER THREE

# LOCAL AND REGIONAL DIAGNOSTIC TOOLS

Can we do better for patients having intact prostates and high-risk disease? We have high expectations that we can do better by incorporating more of the advanced imaging techniques that are now available. With our past published clinical trials, we utilized the USPIO/Feraheme test for many newly diagnosed high-risk patients with Gleason scores 8-10. Only patients with a pacemaker or hemochromatosis would be excluded from having the Feraheme imaging test in the future when it becomes available again, but even those patients may be candidates for contrast-enhanced MRI scans utilizing other agents. As noted, with the third phase of our combined protocol, we routinely treat the pelvic abdominal lymph nodes to eradicate any cancer in those areas. The advances in diagnostic staging have improved our ability to treat prostate cancer at all stages, both local and regional.

## Local Diagnostic Staging Studies

In order to look at local disease burden, we utilize 3D Color-Flow Power Doppler Ultrasound and other state-of-the-art technologies such as Multi-parametric MRI, which can include Dynamic Contrast Enhanced MRI (DCE-MRI), diffusion weighting MRI, and spectrographic MRI.

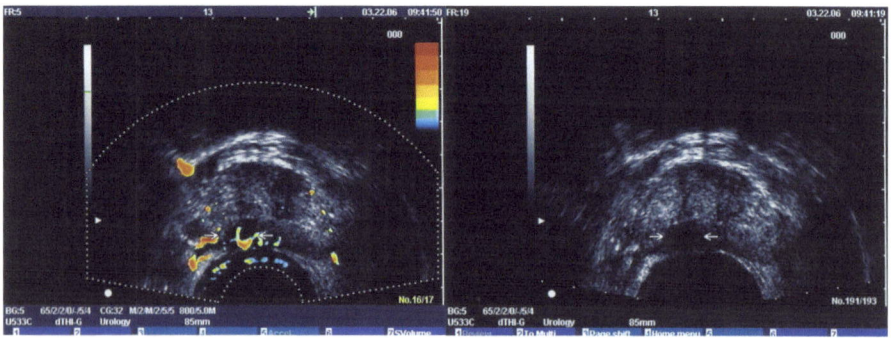

Comparison of Color-Flow Doppler image (left) with conventional gray-scale ultrasound image (right) of the same patient. Note: The bright red areas in the Color-Flow Doppler image reveal the location of suspected cancer sites, which are not visible using gray-scale ultrasound imaging.

## Regional/Distant Diagnostic Staging Studies

In order to look at regional/distant prostate cancer, we utilize a number of advanced staging tests, which include the following:

- Combidex imaging (only currently available in The Netherlands)
- USPIO using Ferumoxytol (Feraheme) nanoparticle (limited availability pending future clinical trials)
- $^{18}$F-FDG fluoride PET/CT
- $^{11}$C–Choline PET/CT–while recently FDA approved, this test has a 15-47% false positivity rate, hence biopsies of abnormalities are still required.
- Carbon 11 acetate Pet/CT–the predictive accuracy of this test is lower than nanoparticle tests, hence biopsies of abnormalities vs. correlative studies appear to be necessary.
- $^{18}$F-Fluciclovine (Axumin) PET/CT-clinical trials in progress.

The nanoparticles used in the Combidex and Feraheme-MRI tests are one millionth of a millimeter. Unfortunately, the Combidex test is only available in the Netherlands and has not yet been granted FDA approval in this country. Likewise, the Feraheme imaging test is awaiting FDA approval, with further clinical trials in the planning stage.

While Feraheme and Combidex are comparable in terms of predictive accuracy, we have found the Ferahema USPIO test superior, with much clearer images that can be fused with our technology in Sarasota.

The $^{18}$F-FDG fluoride PET/CT test is very effective at picking up bone lesions that other tests can miss, and we have also found cancer in the lymph nodes, liver and lungs, especially when the cancer is aggressive (Gleason 8-10). enough to spread to the lungs. The $^{11}$C – Choline PET/CT and the Carbon-11 acetate Pet/CT fusion studies are both useful, but do have a lower predictive accuracy, so patients who are found to have disease by either of these studies may need to be biopsied to confirm the results.

## Combidex Results

A study of the Combidex test published by the *New England Journal of Medicine* in 2003 (*NEJM*: 248, 2491-2498) reported very promising results, summarized as follows:

*33 of 33 patients having prostate lymph node metastasis were successfully identified following lymph node dissection/sampling.*

Another study published in Lancet Oncology in 2008 offered further analysis of Combidex, reporting:

- Positive Predictive Accuracy = 95%
- Negative Predictive Accuracy = 96%

So Combidex has a high predictive accuracy that may allow physicians to proceed to local-regional therapy without performing pelvic lymph node (PLN) dissection.

Below is an example of a Combidex imaging study. The red areas are affected lymph nodes, which are extensive well outside the prostate area. This patient had 46 positive lymph nodes. We treated him and he is doing very well. Treating a patient with this kind of disease spread requires the most sophisticated equipment, both for imaging and delivering the radiation.

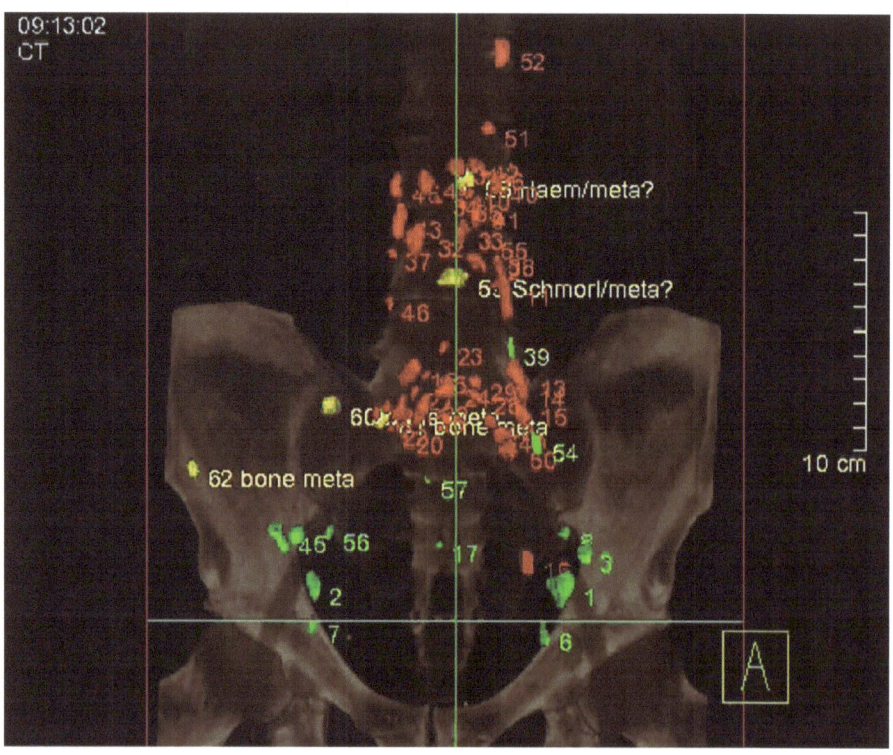

## Tracking the 4th Dimension

In order to properly treat the prostate and especially the lymph nodes, we have to be tracking the 4th dimension, which is motion. We need to be prepared and able to adjust for a patient's motion during treatment, because there will be some organ movement while a patient is undergoing treatment.

Preparation for radiation therapy is a rigorously complex process that involves exact determination of the region to receive treatment and the appropriate dose of radiation. Radiation treatments are precisely designed for each patient, because each man's prostate or prostate bed (if it has not been removed by surgery) and the surrounding organs such as the bladder and rectum are unique in size and shape. A planning session is carried out with the patient several days before treatments begin, and a unique treatment blueprint is mapped out in advance for each patient.

DART utilizes a wide variety of advanced imaging devices. In order to keep the patient in the same position for each daily treatment, we utilize lower-body Vac-Lock and upper-body Wingboard systems, as well as AlignRT skin surface tracking. Daily localization of the target is essential to optimize therapeutic effects since both patient and organ movement may occur. It should be noted that all of the DART Analysis Tools are non-invasive. These daily routines are implemented with comprehensive checklists that are crucial to ensure accurate targeting on a daily basis. We also employ the Varian Exact Couch™ and PortalVision™ with Exact Arm positioning. There are tracking cameras located within the treatment head, which is known as the Exact Arm. If there is more than a millimeter of motion, that will be sensed and a default will come into play.

Once the patient's body is properly aligned, fluoroscopic, computerized tomography and ultrasound imaging techniques are used to visualize the prostate and nearby organs. Our On-Board Imaging Device (OBI), Portal Vision, and 4th generation Cone Beam Helical Tomography add an additional important layer of accuracy checks that ensure a level of precision not dreamed of just five years ago. Even the simple motion of breathing can shift the position of the prostate. But we can track, anticipate and correct for physiologic movement by our special "Respiratory Gating" technology. This is an advanced video tracking technology that allows for real-time monitoring that accounts for patient breathing ("pelvic breathing"). The position of the critical structures will determine where the radiation microbeams should be directed and also the shape of the beams.

The tools described above allow thorough evaluation of the 4th dimension prior to and during treatment to make sure that each microbeam reaches the designated target. Adjustments are constantly made as indicated during treatment. All the components of DART enable us to deliver the right dose to the right target at precisely the right time—each time and every time.

Based on physiological and anatomical changes that occur between individual treatments and during each treatment, our physicians, physicists, dosimetrists, therapists and combination of technical equipment can modulate or alter the original treatment plan to account for these daily changes. This highly integrated approach is the key to DART—intra- and inter-fractional adjustments allowing for the most precise targeting of tumor(s) imaginable.

It should be noted that with DART, not only is the prostate tracked, but also specific areas within the prostate as are all of the surrounding critical tissues (e.g. bladder, rectum, neurovascular bundles, uro-genital diaphram, penile bulb, and proximal areas). Moreover, during the tracking, microbeams are dynamically adjusted to reach their designated target (like "smart missiles"). Typically, patients will receive 8000 to 9000 cGy to the target area, while the urethra will get approximately 20% less. The tumors, depending on where they are located, will receive a higher dose and will be anywhere from 8% to 20% "hotter." There are cases where the dose is 30% or even 40% higher, but those are unusual. And we can do that without any undue side effects.

During DART treatment sessions, beams from several directions converge to form a high-dose target zone, which includes the prostate (when intact) and a variable margin of tissue surrounding the gland. The radiation can be focused on the target area while minimizing the risk of over-radiating the rectum and bladder. We also use SpaceOAR, which creates a temporary space between the rectum and the prostate gland, again sparing healthy tissue. DART utilizes all of the modalities associated with 4-Dimension Image-Guided Intensity Modulated Radiation Therapy (4D IG-IMRT).

# CHAPTER FOUR

# UPDATES ON FERAHEME STATUS AND MRI CONTRAST AGENTS FOR LYMPH NODE IMAGING

Note: The following discussion has been adapted and updated from Dr. Michael Dattoli's September, 2015 presentation for the Prostate Cancer Information Group (P.C.I.G.) of Cincinnati, Ohio.

During the past ten years, the Dattoli Team has participated in a number of clinical trials with Feraheme (USPIO) nanoparticle imaging. For these studies, we partnered with Dr. Stephen Bravo formerly with the Sand Lake Imaging radiology group in Orlando, Florida. With our history of clinical studies undertaken with Dr. Bravo's group, we have accrued enough patients to publish very compelling papers on Feraheme and how effective this approach is in identifying lymph node spread. That research is already completed, and we have what is called "rad path" analysis with those studies, which is used to correlate and determine whether the radiological findings fit the reported pathological diagnosis. Feraheme is used to better enhance what is known as T1 and T2 imaging. When Feraheme is positive for lymph node involvement with specific nodes, biopsies are then used to confirm that finding and demonstrate how effective Feraheme imaging is. We have reported that data and the predictive accuracy is so high that there would be no need for a patient with a positive lymph node that has been detected with Feraheme to have to undergo a lymph node dissection.

After doing many clinical studies utilizing Feraheme for detecting lymph nodes invaded by prostate cancer, Dr. Bravo began to identify certain morphologic changes within lymph nodes with other MRI studies using different contrast media. Dr. Bravo also utilized what is called OptiMark contrast for diffusion weighted nodal imaging. He is also using a similar MRI contrast agent called OptiRay. Choline C-11 PET/CT and the $^{18}$F-Fluciclovine PET/CT scans, which are also advanced imaging techniques for detecting prostate cancer at distant sites (metastatic disease), will also be available. These two modalities involve a fusion approach that combines positron emission tomography (PET) with computerized tomography (CT) scans.

With these additional techniques, we are now able to identify positive lymph nodes and perform biopsies without the use of Feraheme, which has only limited availability as this point. Despite numerous clinical trial presentations that we have reported with Dr. Bravo and his group on Feraheme, in April of 2015 Feraheme was "black boxed" by the FDA for a range of clinical applications. When the FDA black boxes a medication or reagent, it means they are posing a fairly strict warning that this reagent may cause problems, though the reagent continues to be available.

Feraheme has a number of uses in addition to lymph node imaging. It is often administered to patients who are undergoing dialysis, when they are experiencing anemia. Feraheme infusion over time can be used to effectively treat those patients. The FDA also recently granted Feraheme approval for patients suffering from chronic renal failure without being on dialysis. In the case of Feraheme imaging, one NCI trial utilized very high doses of Feraheme, and a number of patients had anaphylactic reactions from which several patients died. Now this was a group of patients who were very ill with life-threatening conditions. Many of them had chronic renal failure and many were on dialysis, so it would be expected that those patients would have reactions with a number of medications. But rather than differentiate Feraheme used at low doses for imagining, the FDA issued a black box on Feraheme across the board, even though there is no danger with the low dose imaging that we utilize in our studies. Using lower dose levels, we have had zero toxicity with our patients. There have been no deaths or anaphylactic reactions. So the most important consideration for the FDA to act on at this point is the low dose levels utilized for Feraheme imaging.

It is important to note that Feraheme is complemented by additional studies that identify prostate cancer spread to parts of the body other than lymph nodes. Because of the fact that when using Feraheme we are basically doing a whole body scan, which is a whole body MRI, and we are also doing a whole body CT scan. Along with those studies, we often utilize a sodium chloride $^{18}$F PET/CT bone scan. So in reality we are testing the whole body.

Feraheme, along with the various MRI contrast agents such as OptiMark and OptiRay, are important additions to our arsenal of imaging techniques. At our center, we utilize lymph node reagents within an all encompassing body scan so the MRI, CT, and PET scans are going to tell us virtually everything about the patient.

Given our long experience working with nanoparticles like Feraheme since the 1990s, we believe that when more radiologists become familiar with the nanoparticle imaging technologies, they are going to want to offer their patients these breakthrough techniques for imaging. For that reason, we plan to offer Feraheme again as soon as the next clinical trial is underway. It is indeed a significant advance that will benefit many patients in the very near future.

# CHAPTER FIVE

# RAISING THE RADIATION DOSE

Stanford University Medical Center researchers treated patients with nodal disease and raised the treatment dose from 66 Gy to 70 Gy, and then upwards to 78 Gy. That amounts to about two more weeks of radiation, which is not very much. But the study showed that biochemical disease free survival improved from 25% with the lower dose patients to 58% with the higher dose patients. Those results are summarized below.

### RT Dose Escalation Studies

**Stanford Post-op Trial**
 4 month ADT, Pelvic Nodal RT
 38 patients median dose 66Gy (ART)
 84 patients median dose 70Gy (ART), 68 patients, median dose 76Gy (SRT)
 Median follow-up > 5 years

**Results:**
 66Gy—25% biochemical freedom at 5 years
 70–76Gy—58% biochemical freedom at 5 years
No increased late toxicities with higher dose.

**Subset Analysis:** most significant prognosticators:
Pre-RT PSA ≤ 1 ng/ml ( p= <0.001) and Negative seminal vesicles (p=0.009)

**Conclusion:** Higher doses increased likelihood of optimal disease free survival.

*King et al, Int J Rad Onc 71: 23-27, 2008*

So increasing the radiation dose more than doubled the successful outcomes with those patients. That was statistically significant and there was no increase in toxicities—no damage to the rectum or bladder, and no increase in erectile dysfunction. So the conclusion is that higher doses increase the chances of patients being cancer free.

A study from Memorial Sloan Kettering also showed a great advantage with high doses. The graph below shows a 45% difference biochemical disease free survival between patients who received low dose (64.8 to 70.2 Gy), intermediate dose (75.6 Gy), and those who received high dose (81 Gy) radiation.

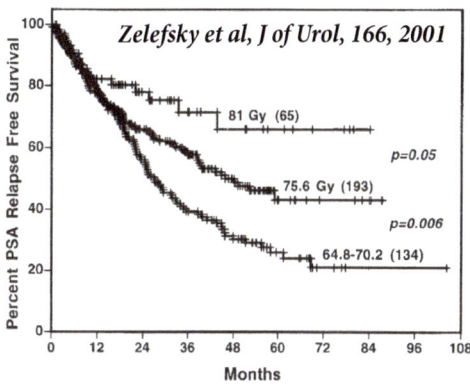

An evidence-based study from M.D. Anderson led by Dr. Deborah Kuban showed the same benefit of treating with even a moderately higher dose escalation. As illustrated by the graph below, with a difference of just 8Gy, at 10 years, the higher dose resulted in 73% biochemical disease free survival versus 50% with the lower dose.

We always treat our patients with the highest dose that can be safely tolerated, but many radiation oncologists still treat their patients with lower doses. Many of those doctors simply don't have the necessary state-of-the-art technology or the expertise to deliver higher doses.

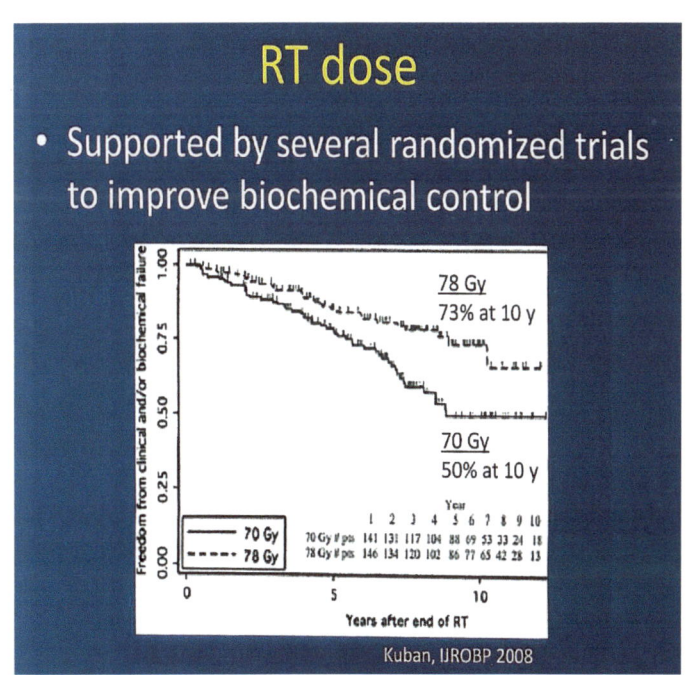

# CHAPTER SIX

# DART AND BIOLOGIC-DIRECTED RADIATION

With all of these imaging modalities that support treatment, we are using what we call "biologic-directed radiation." It is the biologic variables that allow us to selectively target areas of higher tumor burden. These techniques enable us to identify tumor metabolism. Essentially, we fuse all of these studies using different technologies within our computers. The 3D Color-Flow Power Doppler Ultrasound and the Multi-parametric MRI studies help to show us where the cancer is in the prostate. And beyond those, we have modalities like USPIO that allow us to pinpoint where the cancer is outside the prostate. All of these modalities are fused.

DART and Dose De-Modulation/Escalation using these fusion techniques enables us to achieve extraordinary efficacy with our treatment plans. For example, these imaging techniques show us where the urethra is, so we can lessen the dose to the urethra and thereby minimize morbidity when patients have an intact prostate and with patients whose prostates have been removed by surgery.

## DART and Tumor Dose Escalation/Urethral Dose Demodulation Using Fusion Techniques

With the image to the right, we can see exactly the location where the tumor is, so we can give that area a much higher dose to eradicate the cancer. The image of composite radiation for a DART treatment plan shows how

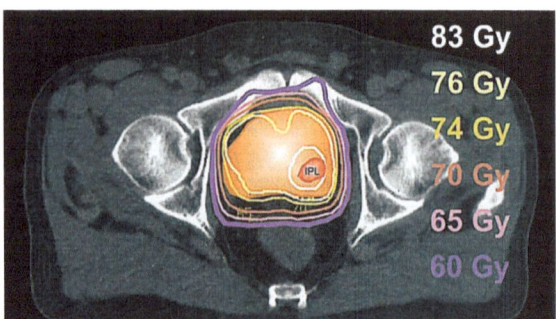

the dose is modulated within the area being treated. The tumor is enclosed by red and receives the highest dose of radiation. This is important because we know that higher doses are most effective at killing cancer, so we can deliver a very high dose accurately to the tumor whether by seeding or with DART or both. The same is true when we know lymph nodes are positive. We can effectively deliver a higher dose to the nodes.

As noted, USPIO is an ultra-small Ferumoxytol nano-particle MRI test that we use to determine if lymph nodes are positive. Suppose a patient goes to Orlando and has a USPIO study that shows he has lymph node disease. What is the best treatment option he has at that point? By fusing the information we get from the portal in Orlando with our technology, as illustrated by the CT/MRI images below, we can see exactly where the lymph nodes are located and we are able to create a precise treatment plan for DART. We can treat a 1-millimeter tumor that was picked up by the Feraheme.

The two images below show para-aortic lymph nodes, which are higher up in the pelvis. These images utilize full-body, Dynamic-contrast MRI technique. The second image actually shows two afffected nodes side by side that we were able to treat successfully with DART. With the high-risk patients that we have discussed in previously published data, we would probably not have treated this high initially. With patients whose initial treatment fails, we will have them undergo the Feraheme or contrast-enhanced MRI, and we often find these positive lymph nodes higher up in the pelvis and also into the abdomen. We will use hormones with these patients along with DART, because the data so far shows an advantage, and we do have ways of mitigating the side effects of hormones.

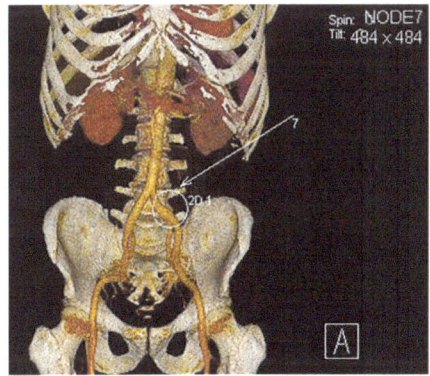
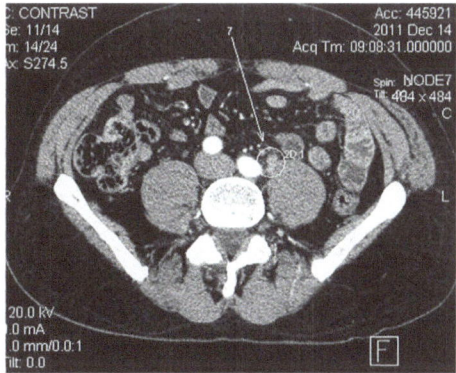

## Treating Abdominal or Para-aortic Nodes

When a patient has lymph node disease in the abdomen para-aortic area, as illustrated in these next images, we can treat the cancer with DART. We can be so precise that only the blue area shown in the top-right image is treated.

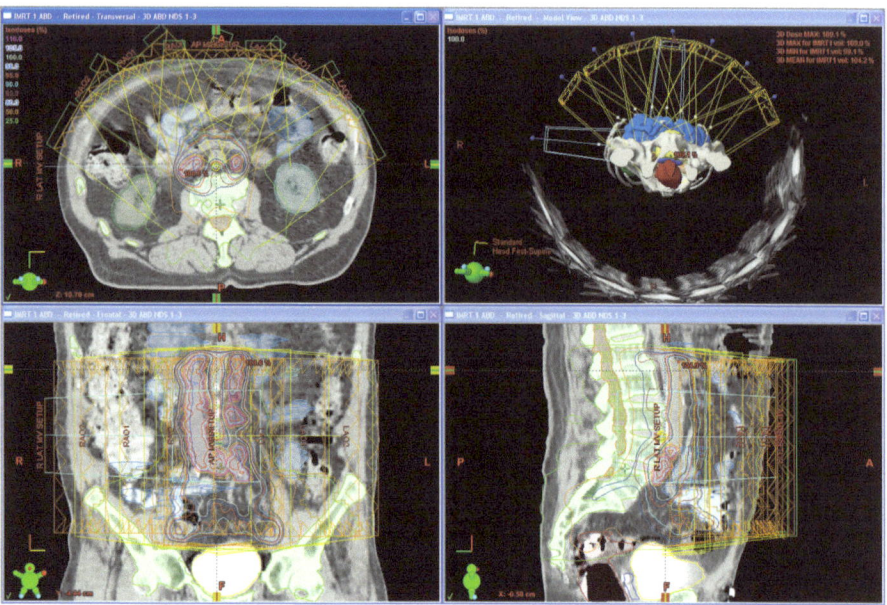

the dose is modulated within the area being treated. The tumor is enclosed by red and receives the highest dose of radiation. This is important because we know that higher doses are most effective at killing cancer, so we can deliver a very high dose accurately to the tumor whether by seeding or with DART or both. The same is true when we know lymph nodes are positive. We can effectively deliver a higher dose to the nodes.

As noted, USPIO is an ultra-small Ferumoxytol nano-particle MRI test that we use to determine if lymph nodes are positive. Suppose a patient goes to Orlando and has a USPIO study that shows he has lymph node disease. What is the best treatment option he has at that point? By fusing the information we get from the portal in Orlando with our technology, as illustrated by the CT/MRI images below, we can see exactly where the lymph nodes are located and we are able to create a precise treatment plan for DART. We can treat a 1-millimeter tumor that was picked up by the Feraheme.

The two images below show para-aortic lymph nodes, which are higher up in the pelvis. These images utilize full-body, Dynamic-contrast MRI technique. The second image actually shows two afffected nodes side by side that we were able to treat successfully with DART. With the high-risk patients that we have discussed in previously published data, we would probably not have treated this high initially. With patients whose initial treatment fails, we will have them undergo the Feraheme or contrast-enhanced MRI, and we often find these positive lymph nodes higher up in the pelvis and also into the abdomen. We will use hormones with these patients along with DART, because the data so far shows an advantage, and we do have ways of mitigating the side effects of hormones.

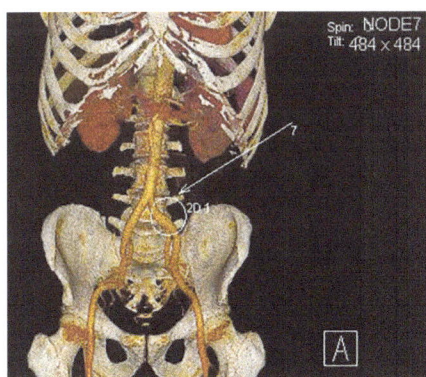
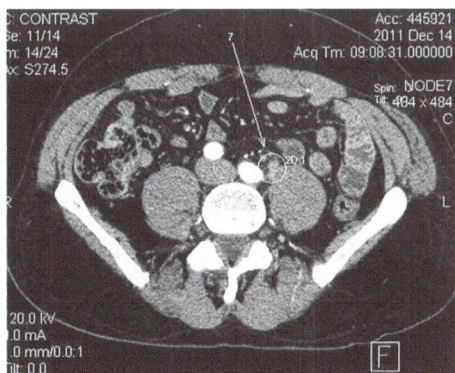

## Treating Abdominal or Para-aortic Nodes

When a patient has lymph node disease in the abdomen para-aortic area, as illustrated in these next images, we can treat the cancer with DART. We can be so precise that only the blue area shown in the top-right image is treated.

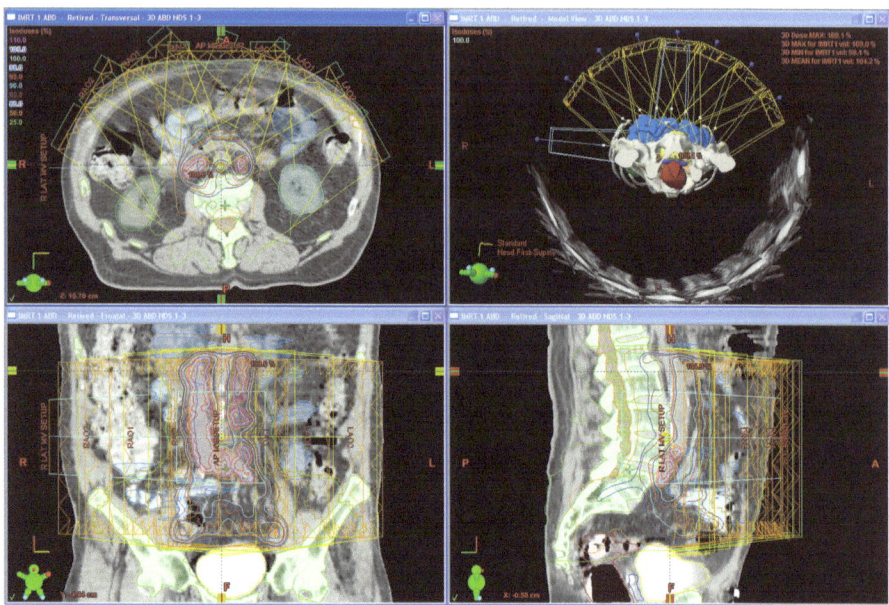

# CHAPTER SEVEN

# COMPARING PRIMARY TREATMENT OPTIONS FOR HIGH RISK PATIENTS

## Surgery versus Combination Protocol Radiotherapy

With high-risk patients, the most effective way to avoid lymph node disease is to treat the pelvic and abdominal lymph nodes with the primary treatment. Radiotherapy can treat lymph notes, while radical surgery only removes the prostate gland and can only, at best sample lymph nodes (which is even further limited using robotic approaches). As such, we do not believe that radical surgery (open or robotic) should be used to treat high-risk patients when a significant number of those men will be shown to have lymph node disease.

With intermediate and high-risk patients (PSA greater than 10, Gleason 7 to 10, clinical state equal to or greater than T2b), the data shows that these patients have a high risk for biochemical failure after radical prostatectomy. Indeed, it is with the higher risk groups that the results obtained with surgery have deteriorated to the point of being woefully unacceptable. As illustrated by the three graphs below, the lack of any plateau (leveling off) in the disease-free survival curves of surgery patients with a pre-treatment PSA above 10 and/or a Gleason score of 7 or higher is especially striking coming from a leading institution like Johns Hopkins Medical Center (see Figures 1-2).

The bottom line on radical surgery becomes all the more stark when we look at the most recent long-term cure rates with high risk patients from Johns Hopkins. That series, utilizing Dr. Patrick Walsh's long term data, (Pierorazio PM, et al., Urology. 2010 Mar 27) reports, "The results of our study have shown that 80% of the men with Gleason sum 8-10 who undergo RP will have experienced biochemical recurrence by 15 years."

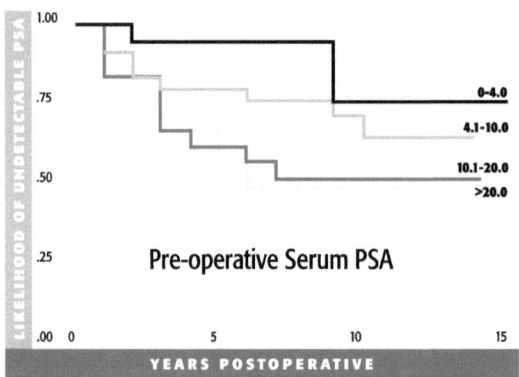

**FIGURE 1**—Likelihood of biochemical failure (rising PSA) by pre-operative serum (Khan MA Partin AW, The Oncologist, Vil. No. 3, 259-269, June 2003). Data derived from the series by Dr. Patrick Walsh, Johns Hopkins Hospital, 1982-2001 (Figures 8–9). COURTESY OF THE ONCOLOGIST

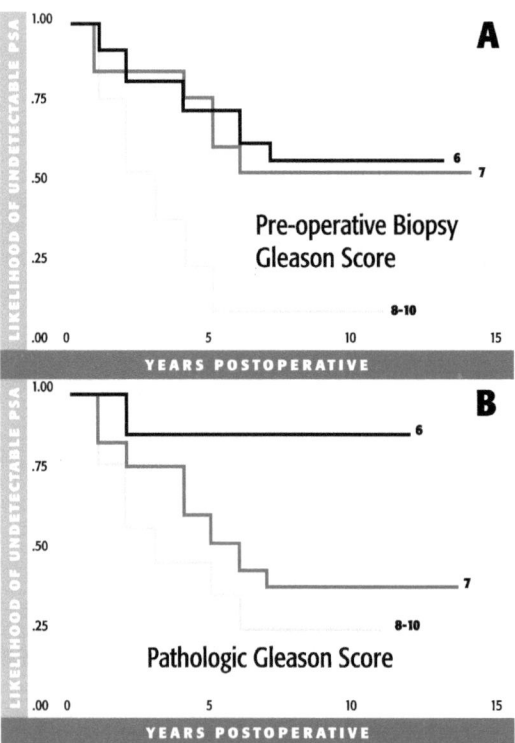

**FIGURE 2**—The likelihood of biochemical failure (rising PSA) by pre-operative biopsy Gleason score (A) and by pathologic Gleason score (B). COURTESY OF THE ONCOLOGIST

To put it another way, at 15 years for high-risk patients undergoing radical surgery, the success rate is only 20% in the very best hands at one of the leading centers of excellence. Based on data like that, we encourage patients to think long and hard before making the choice to have radical surgery, whether carried out by hand or robotically.

The two graphs in Figures 1 and 2 (A and B) were adapted from a 2003 study in The Oncologist, with our results inserted for comparison. The graphs compare surgery with the Dattoli combination protocol of brachytherapy and external radiation therapy. Brachytherapy combined with external radiation therapy versus surgery, as primary therapies for high-risk patients. Patients are stratified by PSA greater than 20 in Figure 1 and by biopsy and pathologic Gleason score in Figure 2 (A and B). These high-risk post-surgical patients frequently come to our center after they have experienced treatment failure as indicated by rising PSA values. They turn to us for salvage radiation.

Given all the evidence-based data we have for high-risk prostate cancer, external radiation plus brachytherapy (with or without hormones) appears to be superior to radical prostatectomy. And with 74% successful outcomes with high-risk patients with PSA values greater than 20, we believe some of those patients had cancer just outside the top of the pelvic treatment field that we missed at that time. By expanding the treatment using USPIO data, we are now able to treat those men more effectively, greatly increasing the likelihood that even high-risk patients will be free from lymph node positive disease.

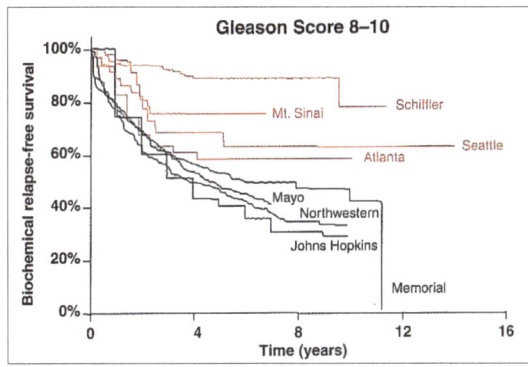

**Survival After Brachytherapy vs Prostatectomy, by Gleason Score**—Biochemical relapse-free survival among patients with Gleason score 8–9 treated definitively with brachytherapy and supplemental external-beam radiation (red) or radical prostatectomy (black). *Oncology*, Vol 22, No 9, 2008

It should be noted that combining brachytherapy with supplemental external radiotherapy does not have a negative impact on side effects. Two randomized studies have compared brachytherapy alone with brachytherapy combined with external radiation. One study actually showed that the combination therapy caused fewer long-term side effects than seed implants alone (Ghaley et al, *Int J. Rad Onc*, Vol 55, 2003). The other study showed that 5-year biochemical disease-free survival is improved 21% by combining brachytherapy with external radiation versus

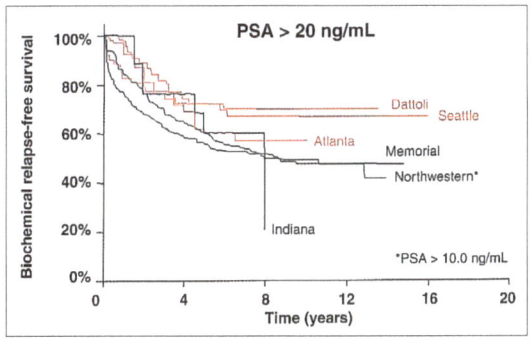

**Survival After Brachytherapy vs Prostatectomy, by PSA Level**—Biochemical relapse-free survival among patients with prostate-specific antigen (PSA) >20 ng/mL treated definitively with brachytherapy and supplemental external-beam radiation (red) or radical prostatectomy (black). *Oncology*, Vol 22, No 9, 2008

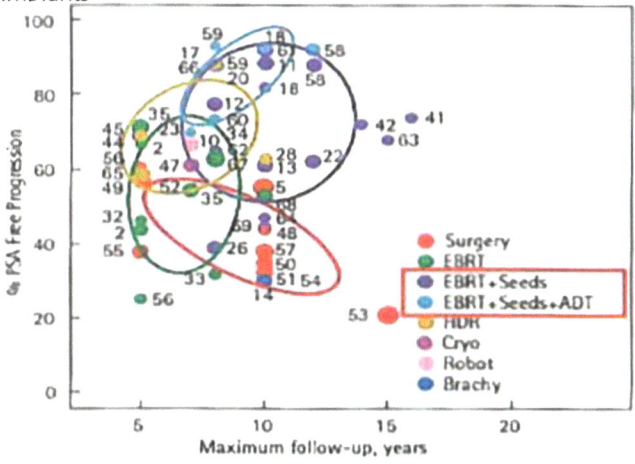

brachytherapy alone (*U of Chicago, Jani et al, Urology, Vol 67, Issue 5, May 2006, pages 1007-1011*).

The graph at right illustrates the results of a recent depth analysis conducted by a research team led by the late Dr. Peter Grimm of Seattle. These researchers reviewed more than 25,000 studies published from 2000 to 2012 that reported on the currently available primary treatments, including radical surgery (open and robotic), external radiation alone, brachytherapy alone, brachytherapy and external radiation combined, cryosurgery, hormonal therapy alone and combined with surgery and radiation, and high dose rate radiation. The studies reported treatment outcomes with the various modalities. An expert panel of 28 leading researchers participated in analyzing the results (Grimm P, et al, *BJU Int.* 2012 Feb; 109 Suppl 1:22-9).

As illustrated by the graph, these researchers found that high-risk patients treated with brachytherapy combined with external radiation had the greatest likelihood of being cancer free at up to 15 years. Our own study was in agreement at 15-years (and later at 16-years) and was indicated in the graph as study #41 (*Dattoli, et al, Journal of Oncology, July 2010*). A full summary of our 16-year series is presented in Appendix A. To date, we have reported the most successful long-term results in the world for intermediate and high-risk patients.

# APPENDIX A

# A SUMMARY OF THE 16-YEAR DATA

The following summary is based on a Dattoli series that was first presented at an American Society of Clinical Oncology meeting (February, 2009), and subsequently published in the *Journal of Oncology* (Dattoli M, Wallner K True L, Bostwick D, Cash J, Sorace, R, Long-term Outcomes for Patients with Prostate Cancer having Intermediate and High-risk Disease, treated with Brachytherapy and Supplemental External Beam Radiotherapy, J Oncol. 2010; pii: 471375. Epub 2010 Aug 18). The summary also draws on an earlier published series (Dattoli M, et al., *Urology,* 2007 Feb; 69(2):334-337).

The bottom line in our studies is that these are patients who were at high risk, with a high likelihood of extra-prostatic extension (cancer that has spread outside the prostate gland). These patients were treated with 3D-Conformal Radiation (which was the state-of-the-art approach prior to the IMRT era) followed by seed implantation, with large margins. The study was by a single author-practitioner doing the implants, but the biochemical data was independently reviewed by the University of Washington, and all the slides were re-reviewed by the University of Washington, which adds an element of security to the data. Clinical stage was not included because the doctors at the University of Washington couldn't perform a digital rectal exam on these patients due to geographical distance. These results will serve as a baseline for comparison with the alternative treatment options.

It should be noted that DART is far more precise and delivers a significantly higher dose than 3D-CRT. A number of studies have shown that higher doses greatly increase the likelihood of patients being cancer-free after treatment. At our center, we have been employing DART in our combined protocol with brachytherapy since 2005, and during the intervening years, we are confident that our results have further improved even since we first reported our 16-year series.

## Materials and Methods
321 Consecutive Patients treated by one author (M.D.)—157 intermediate risk and 164 high risk.

## Selection Criteria
NCCN Guidelines

## Radiation Treatment Regimen
- 3D-CRT Dose: 4140cGy Median (Range 39 Gy–54 Gy)
- Pd-103 Dose: 8000-9000 Minimum Peripheral Dose (pre-NIST-99)
- Source Strength: 1.4 mCi Median (Range 1.1-1.6 mCi)
- Clinical Pd-103 Target Volume: extended 0.5 – 1.0 cm, antero-laterally to the TRUS prostate margin
- Patients were followed at 3, 6 and 12 months, and every 6-12 months thereafter
- Definition of biochemical success: PSA <0.2 ng/ml, nadir +2 and ASTRO Consensus Definition (3 consecutive PSA rises)
- Follow-up saturation prostate biopsies were performed on all failing patients
- Biochemical data independently re-reviewed and analyzed by Kent Wallner, MD (Univ. of Washington)
- Original biopsy slides re-reviewed by Lawrence True, MD (Univ. of Washington)
- Clinical stage was not included in final data analysis to reduce subjectivity

## Patient Characteristics
- Mean PSA 19.4 (1.6–147)
- Median PSA 16.4
- 218 Patients had Gleason Score 7-10
- 203 Patients had PSA > 10
- 79 Patients had elevated PAPs
- 141 Patients had Clinical Stage T2C
- 127 Patients had Clinical Stage T3

## Follow-up
- 16 year actuarial, Median 10.3 years
- 143 Patients received a median of 4 months neo-adjuvant or adjuvant therapy

# APPENDIX A: SUMMARY OF THE 16-YEAR DATA

## Results

➢ PAP was the strongest predictor of failure (p= 0.0001), followed by Gleason Score (p< 0.001) and PSA (p=0.03)

➢ Hormones conferred no survival advantage (p=0.4) although patients receiving hormones had the most adverse features (Stage T3, Gleason 8-10, and elevated PAP results)

➢ 82% overall actuarial freedom from biochemical progress at 16 years using strict PSA nadir of <0.2 ng/ml (Freedom from failure calculated by method of Kaplan-Meier. Difference between groups were determined by the log rank or students' t-test) (86% cancer specific survival; 89% intermediate and 74% high risk)

➢ The absolute risk of failure fell to 1% beyond 5 years after treatment

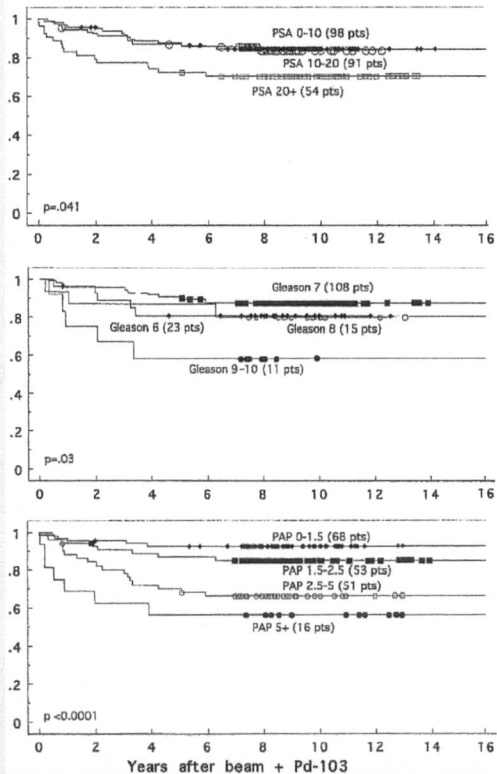

These three graphs show the freedom of biographical progression of the disease out to 16 years stratified by PSA, Gleason Score, and PAP.

➢ Treatment morbidity was limited to RTOG grade 1-2 symptoms. No patients experienced grade 3-4 toxicity. (One patient who had both a TURP and TUIP developed low-volume stress incontinence.) No patient developed rectal ulceration

➢ All failing patients underwent saturation prostatic biopsies. There were no pathologically documented local failures

## Conclusions

➢ Patients having high risk prostate cancer may enjoy long-term biochemical freedom even when using strict PSA nadirs

➤ Morbidity has been very acceptable
➤ Despite the aggressive nature of this study group, no local failures have been documented
➤ It is encouraging that the failure rate decreased to near zero with follow-up beyond 5 years
➤ These results appear superior to surgery, aggressive external beam radiotherapy (including full course IMRT ± hormones, protons/neutrons or combined radiation methods using other isotopes ± hormones) in this high risk group
➤ We attribute these exceedingly favorable results, in part, to our effort to achieve wide brachytherapy treatment margins. This is accomplished by using highly peripheral and extraprostatic source placement designed with concave ends to reduce "source migration"
➤ PD-103 appears to be the isotope best suited for high-risk cancers

This graph shows the likelihood of subsequent bio-chemical failure versus years after treatment. These results are encouraging because as time goes on fewer and fewer patients experience biochemical failure, indicated by a PSA greater than 0.2.

# APPENDIX B

# DATTOLI LYMPH NODE IMAGING STUDIES

The following abstract was presented at two medical conferences in February, 2018, the Annual Symposium on Clinical Interventional Oncology (CIO) and the Genitourinary Cancers Symposium cosponsored by the American Society of Clinical Oncology (ASCO), the American Society for Radiation Oncology (ASTRO), and the Society of Urologic Oncology (SUO).

## Efficacy of Feraheme as Lymphatic Contrast Agent in Prostate Cancer

*Dattoli MJ, Bravo SM, Kaplon DM, Hayes M, Osorio A,
Dycus PM, Bostwick D, Kaminski JM*

**BACKGROUND:** Ferumoxytol (Feraheme), a ferromagnetic nanoparticle with lymphotrophic biokinetics, is delivered to lymph nodes via normal macrophages. MRI suppresses normal lymph nodes containing Feraheme. Objective is to validate the agent's safety and efficacy in finding lymph node positivity in prostate cancer (PCa).

**METHODS:** Nonrandomized prospective evaluation of 178 consecutive PCa patients (pts) at high risk for prostate lymph node spread were enrolled 2/13-3/15. All received IV Feraheme. 177 received infusion of 6/mg/kg given over 20 minutes. One pt received 3 mg/kg infusion. T2 MEDIC and T2* sequence imaging of the abdomen and pelvis, performed 24 hours later. Images were reviewed by 2 board certified radiologists with same interpretations, blinded to clinical and histopath information (pre-MRI TNM stage, PSA or Gleason score). Lymph nodes were deemed abnormal if they did not suppress after Feraheme infusion (group 1, 94 patients). Lymph nodes were deemed suspicious by MRI if suppressed and met usual size criteria with high signal intensity on DWI and decreased ADC map values and morphologic features (group 2, 84 pts). 83 group 1 pts had CT biopsies (77 pelvis, 6 retroperitoneum); 11 pts had open PLND. 382 lymph nodes were sampled. 76 group 2 patients had CT biopsies (73 pelvis, 3 retroperitoneum); 9 pts had open PLND. 340 lymph nodes were sampled. Rad-path correlation was performed. Resected nodes were stained; reviewed by a single pathologist with no knowledge of MRI findings. The histo-path results for each node were cataloged for later MRI comparison.

**RESULTS:** 90 group 1 pts (96%) proved metastatic PCa; 4 pts (4%) were normal. 68 group 1 pts (77%) contained malignant lymph nodes not meeting usual imaging criteria for malignancy. 39 group 2 pts showed metastatic PCa; 46 pts (53%) were normal. One group 2 pt experienced an allergic reaction with hives; infusion ceased at 3mg/kg; pt treated to full resolution with 50 mg IV Benadryl.

**CONCLUSION:** Feraheme can be used to evaluate for lymphatic dissemination of metastatic disease in PCa patients, with a lower limit of resolution of focal lymph node metastases of 2-3 mm. Improved resolution brings implications for therapeutic radiation planning in setting of newly diagnosed or recurrent/metastatic PCa. Toxicity was very acceptable at 6mg/kg. Feraheme may play a significant role as a lymphatic contrast agent in the early dissemination of lymphatic metastatic disease.

---

At the time of this writing, the following abstract is scheduled for presentation at the Genitourinary Cancers Symposium (February 13-15, 2020) co-sponsored by the American Society of Clinical Oncology (ASCO), the American Society for Radiation Oncology (ASTRO), and the Society of Urologic Oncology (SUO). This retrospective study on USPIO imaging (utilizing the Combidex contrast agent) and treating lymph node positive prostate cancer was conducted by the Dattoli Cancer & Brachytherapy Research Institute in collaboration with the Helen Diller Family Comprehensive Cancer Center at the University of California San Francisco, and the Radboud University Medical Center, Nijmegen, the Netherlands.

Molecular imaging techniques including F18-PET, Ga-68-PSMA-PET and high-resolution MRIs have revolutionized the staging and management of patients with high risk and oligometastatic prostate cancer (Harmon, J. Nuc Med, 2017). However, the detection threshold of these methods is limited, particularly for early lymph node metastases (Joniau, Eur Urol, 2013). Recent data suggests that aggressive treatment of oligometastatic prostate cancer (limited number of metastases) may prolong survival in selected patients (Ost, JCO, 2018). This study evaluates the use of Ultra-Small Super-Paramagnetic Iron Oxide (USPIO) MRIs, which is potentially even more sensitive than PET imaging, as a technique for detection and irradiation of involved lymph nodes.

# Radiotherapy guided by ultra small superparamagnetic iron oxide (USPIO)-contrast MRI staging for patients with advanced or recurrent prostate cancer.

**Yun Rose Li** – *Department of Radiation Oncology and Helen Diller Family Comprehensive Cancer Center, University of California San Francisco, San Francisco, CA, USA.*

**Michael J. Dattoli** – *Dattoli Cancer Center and Brachytherapy Research Institute, Sarasota, FL, USA.*

**Jelle Barentsz** – *Department of Radiology and Nuclear Medicine, RadboudUMC, Nijmegen, the Netherlands.*

**Mack Roach III** – *Department of Radiation Oncology and Helen Diller Family Comprehensive Cancer Center, University of California San Francisco, San Francisco, CA, USA.*

**BACKGROUND:** Aggressive treatment of oligometastatic PC may prolong survival in selected patients. USPIO-contrast MRI is potentially more sensitive in detecting early lymph node (LN) metastases than PET.

**METHODS:** This retrospective study explores the safety and utility of USPIO-guided RT in 69 patients with advanced/recurrent PC treated at 2 US institutions. All SPIO-MRIs were completed at RadboudUMC and interpreted by expert radiologists. Age, Stage, Gleason score, PSA, prior therapy, duration of androgen-deprivation (ADT), cause of death, details of RT, and adverse events (AEs) were collected by chart review. Biochemical recurrence (BCR) was defined as PSA Nadir plus 2.0 (RT) or PSA > 0.2 (radical prostatectomy, RP). Patients received external beam radiation (RT) to involved nodal basins (+/- prostate/prostate bed) with either a simultaneous integrated or sequential boost to USPIO(+) nodes. All patients received >6 months of ADT. Overall (OS) and BCR free-survival (BCRFS) were calculated using Cox-PH models in R.

**RESULTS:** Between 2007-18, 69 patients with de novo or recurrent PC were found to have USPIO(+) LNs and received USPIO-guided RT; median age was 62. The majority of patients presented after BCR following RP (N = 28), definitive RT (N = 27) or RP and post-op RT (N = 6). Prior to USPIO-MRI, 20/69 patients had cN1 disease based on abdominal-pelvic CT/MRI, Bone Scan, Prostascint-scan, and F18 Choline, Axumin or PSMA PET/CT. The mean(median)USPIO(+) LNs was 5.2(3) Range = [1-32]. Patients had (+)pelvic (95%), para-aortic (43%), and/or peri-rectal LNs (19%). At median follow up of 29.5(44.6) Range = [5-127] months, OS was 58/69 (84%) and 11/11 patients died of PC. At last follow up, 40 patients remained BCR-free (BCRFS not reached). The median time to BCR (N = 29) was 25.9 months after USPIO-guided RT. For patients with follow-up imaging, recurrences were predominantly out-of-field (outside of elective LN fields or in osseous sites). No patients experienced > CTCAE grade 2 AEs.

**CONCLUSION:** In this cohort of 69 patients with predominantly recurrent PC, USPIO-directed RT was well-tolerated, feasible and resulted in encouraging biochemical control rates.

# APPENDIX C

# DR. DATTOLI ON TREATING METASTATIC DISEASE

When prostate cancer spreads beyond its original site and is no longer locally confined to the prostate gland—a process called metastasis—it marks a significant turning point in the disease for patients. For many, this diagnosis can feel overwhelming, as metastatic cancer has historically been considered incurable. However, the landscape of advanced prostate cancer treatment has evolved significantly over the past two decades thanks to technological progress and our growing knowledge of the disease. Today, there are innovative strategies that offer patients hope for improved survival while maintaining their quality of life.

Our current understanding of metastatic prostate cancer and modern approaches to treatment that have redefined what is possible for those facing this potentially life-threatening diagnosis.

## Understanding Metastatic Prostate Cancer

Metastatic prostate cancer occurs when cancer cells spread from the prostate to other parts of the body, most commonly the lymph nodes, bones, lungs, and liver. Historically, metastatic prostate cancer was treated with systemic therapies alone—such as androgen deprivation therapy (ADT) and chemotherapy—aimed at controlling cancer throughout the body. However, these approaches often left persistent cancer cells in the prostate gland itself or in localized metastatic sites, which had since become resistant to systemic agents.

As a result, these remaining cancer cells often progress and spread, leading to problems within the prostate region itself. These cancer cells are also left to colonize distant sites such as the lymph nodes, bone, lungs and liver.

## A Shift in Perspective

For decades, the prevailing belief was that treating the primary tumor in cases of metastasis was futile. However, emerging evidence has challenged this view. Research now suggests that treating the prostate gland – even in the context of metastasis–can influence outcomes by reducing tumor burden and potentially slowing or preventing further spread.

One of the most intriguing concepts in this field is that of the *abscopal effect*. This phenomenon describes how local treatments like radiation therapy not only target tumors at their primary site of origin but also stimulate systemic immune responses that shrink untreated tumors elsewhere in the body. This discovery opened new doors for integrating local and systemic therapies for effectively managing metastatic prostate cancer.

## The Evidence: Key Clinical Trials

Several landmark studies have reshaped our understanding of metastatic prostate cancer treatment:

### 1. The STAMPEDE Trial (2016)

This large, randomized trial demonstrated that adding radiation therapy to systemic treatments (such as ADT) provided a significant survival benefit for men with metastatic prostate cancer, and especially for those having low-volume metastatic disease. The study showed that targeting the primary tumor with radiation could improve outcomes even when metastases were present (James, ND et al, Addition of docetaxel, zoledronic acid, or both to first-line long-term hormone therapy in prostate cancer (STAMPEDE): survival results from an adaptive, multiarm, multistage, platform randomized controlled trial; Lancet, 2016 Mar 19;387(10024):1163-77).

### 2. The HORRAD Trial

This clinical trial explored the benefits of combining radiation therapy with ADT specifically for men with bone metastases. The results demonstrated beneficial outcomes in patients having low-volume skeletal metastases, although even treating high-volume disease with this combined approach was associated with several superior clinical and radiographic endpoints (Boevé LMS, et al, Prostate Cancer-related Events in Patients with Synchronous Metastatic Hormone-sensitive Prostate Cancer Treated with Androgen Deprivation Therapy with and Without Concurrent Radiation Therapy to the Prostate; Data from the HORRAD Trial. Eur Urol. 2024 Sep 19:S0302-2838(24)02593-4).

## 3. Oligometastatic Disease Concept

A concept introduced in 1995 by University of Chicago researchers Weichselbaum and Hellman, who coined the term "oligometastases," referring to cases where cancer has spread to a limited number of distant sites (typically up to five) outside the prostate. Studies suggest that patients with oligometastatic disease may achieve long-term complete remissions—or even cure—through aggressive local treatments targeting *both* the primary tumor and metastatic sites (Oligometastases. Hellman S, Weichselbaum RR. J Clin Oncol. 1995 Jan;13(1):8-10.

# Modern Treatment Strategies: A Multi-Pronged Approach

The treatment of advanced prostate cancer now often involves a combination of therapies tailored to each patient's disease characteristics. Below are key components of this multi-pronged approach:

## 1. Treating the Primary Tumor

Radiation therapy directed at the prostate gland remains a cornerstone of definitive treatment for localized prostate cancer. By reducing the tumor burden at its source, this approach can delay progression and minimize complications such as urinary obstruction or pelvic pain. Recent clinical trials have validated the use of local radiation to the prostate even in the metastatic setting as well.

## 2. Metastasis-Directed Therapy

Advances in imaging technologies like PSMA PET scans have made it possible to precisely identify metastatic sites early in their development. This has enabled targeted radiation to treat these sites directly—a strategy known as metastasis-directed therapy (MDT).

• MDT can be particularly effective for patients with oligometastatic disease.
• Precision radiation techniques such as Intensity Modulated Radiation Therapy (IMRT) and Stereotactic Body Radiotherapy (SBRT) are used to deliver highly focused doses to metastatic lesions while sparing surrounding healthy tissue.

## 3. Systemic Therapies

Systemic treatments remain essential for controlling widespread disease. They include the following:

• **Androgen Deprivation Therapy (ADT):** In its multivarious forms, ADT represents the historic foundation of systemic therapy for prostate cancer.

• **Androgen Receptor Pathway Inhibitors:** Drugs like enzalutamide (Xtandi), apalutamide (Erleada), abiraterone (Zytiga), and darolutamide (Nubeqa®) enhance ADT by blocking testosterone signaling more effectively than ADT alone.

- **Chemotherapy:** Docetaxel or cabazitaxel are often used in combination with hormone therapy.
- **Radioligand Therapy:** Agents like Xofigo (radium-223) and Pluvicto (lutetium-177 PSMA) deliver targeted radiation directly to cancer cells.
- **Immunotherapy:** Sipuleucel-T (Provenge) is an FDA-approved vaccine-based immunotherapy for advanced prostate cancer, often referred to as "designer immunotherapy."
- **Molecularly Targeted Therapies:** Genomic profiling can identify actionable mutations for personalized treatments using PARP inhibitors or monoclonal antibodies.
- **Precision Medicine:** The role of state-of-the-art imaging technologies has revolutionized how metastatic prostate cancer is detected and managed.
  - PSMA PET Imaging provides unparalleled accuracy in identifying even small metastases.
  - Combidex/USPIO Nanoparticle Imaging is used to detect the earliest microscopic lymph node involvement.

These tools allow clinicians to stratify patients into low-volume versus high-volume metastatic disease categories and tailor treatment plans accordingly.

## Real-World Success Stories

At the Dattoli Cancer Center, these advanced concepts have been applied with remarkable success. Over the past two decades, many patients with advanced metastatic prostate cancer have achieved long-term complete remissions—many remaining cancer-free for well over 10 years—through aggressive yet precise protocols that are safe.

### Key elements of our approach include:

- Dynamic Adaptive Radiation Therapy (DART), which is an extremely precise form of external beam radiation used to target both the prostate and regional lymph nodes.
- Metastasis-directed DART for skeletal or visceral metastases.
- Integration of systemic therapies such as ADT and androgen receptor inhibitors.
- Use of radioligand therapies (e.g., Xofigo, Pluvicto) and immunotherapies (e.g., Provenge).
- Molecular profiling to guide precision medicine strategies.

Toxicity profiles have been very mild, making these treatments both effective and well-tolerated by our patients, especially compared to chemotherapy.

## The Path Forward

The treatment paradigm for metastatic prostate cancer has shifted dramatically from one of palliative care alone to one that embraces long-term curative potential.

A comprehensive strategy combining local therapies, metastasis-directed interventions, and systemic agents offers new hope for extending survival and improving quality of life.

For patients diagnosed with metastatic prostate cancer today—including both newly diagnosed patients and those who experience recurrence—there is no longer a single path forward but rather a spectrum of options tailored to individual needs and disease characteristics. By leveraging advances in imaging, precision medicine, and multidisciplinary care, we are entering an era where even advanced stages of this disease can be managed with much optimism about potential success in the near-term.

Toxicity profiles have been very mild, making these treatments both effective and well-tolerated by our patients, especially compared to chemotherapy.

## The Path Forward

The treatment paradigm for metastatic prostate cancer has shifted dramatically from one of palliative care alone to one that embraces long-term curative potential.

A comprehensive strategy combining local therapies, metastasis-directed interventions, and systemic agents offers new hope for extending survival and improving quality of life.

For patients diagnosed with metastatic prostate cancer today—including both newly diagnosed patients and those who experience recurrence—there is no longer a single path forward but rather a spectrum of options tailored to individual needs and disease characteristics. By leveraging advances in imaging, precision medicine, and multidisciplinary care, we are entering an era where even advanced stages of this disease can be managed with much optimism about potential success in the near-term.

# APPENDIX D

# GLOSSARY OF MEDICAL TERMS

**3D-CRT (3-Dimensional Conformal Radiation Therapy):** *See Conformal Radiotherapy.*

**5-alpha reductase (5-AR):** an enzyme that converts testosterone to dihydrotestosterone (DHT).

**Adenocarcinoma:** A cancer originating in glandular tissue. Prostate cancer is classified as adenocarcinoma of the prostate.

**Adjuvant:** An additional treatment used to increase the effectiveness of the primary therapy. Radiation therapy and hormonal therapy are often used as adjuvant treatments following a radical prostatectomy. Compare Neoadjuvant.

**Agonist:** A chemical substance that combines with a receptor on a cell and initiates an activity or reaction. *See LHRH analogs.*

**Algorithm:** A step-by-step procedure for solving a problem or accomplishing some end, especially by a computer.

**Analog:** A man-made chemical compound that is structurally similar to one produced naturally by the body. *See LHRH analogs.*

**Anastomotic stricture:** narrowing, usually by scarring, of an anastomotic suture line.

**Androgen:** A hormone that produces male characteristics. *See testosterone.*

**Androgen ablation therapy:** A therapy designed to inhibit the body's production of testosterones.

**Androgen-dependent cells:** Prostate cancer cells which are nourished by male hormones and therefore are capable of being destroyed by hormone deprivation (also known as androgen-sensitive cells).

**Androgen-independent cells:** Prostate cancer cells which are not dependent on male hormones and therefore do not respond to hormonal therapy (also known as androgen-insensitive cells).

**Anesthetic:** A drug that produces general or local loss of physical sensations, particularly pain. A "spinal" is the injection of a local anesthetic into the area surrounding the spinal cord.

**Aneuploid:** Having an abnormal number of chromosomes, as revealed by ploidy analysis. Aneuploid prostate cancer cells tend not to respond well to androgen deprivation therapy (ADT).

**Angiogenesis:** The body's formation of new blood vessels. Some anti-cancer drugs work by blocking angiogenesis, thus preventing blood from reaching and nourishing a tumor.

**Antagonist:** A chemical substance in the body that acts to reduce the physiological activity of another chemical substance.

**Antiandrogens:** Drugs such as Casodex that block the activity of androgens produced by the adrenal glands at the cellular receptor sites. Androgens can block or neutralize the effects of testosterone and DHT on prostate cancer cells.

**Antibody:** A protein produced by the body that counteracts the toxic effects of a foreign substance, organism, or disease within the body.

**Antigen:** A foreign substance such as a virus or bacterium that causes an immune response or the formation of an antibody.

**Antineoplastic:** Inhibits growth and proliferation of cancer cells.

**Antioxidants:** Any substances which delay the process of oxidation in the body.

**Apoptosis:** The normal molecular mechanism which governs the life span of cells so that they die in a very organized way. Cancerous cells are resistant to normal apoptosis.

**Benign:** A non-cancerous condition. *See also Benign Prostatic Hypertrophy.*

**Benign Prostatic Hypertrophy (BPH):** Also called Benign Prostatic Hyperplasia, BPH is a non-cancerous condition of the prostate that results in a growth of tumorous tissue and increase in the size of the prostate.

**Biopsy:** A procedure involving the removal of tissue from the body of the patient. Removed tissue is typically examined microscopically by a pathologist in order to make a precise diagnosis of the patient's condition.

**Bone scan:** An imaging technique used to detect bone metastases, which appear as "hot spots" on the film. It is far more sensitive than the conventional x-ray.

**BPH:** *See Benign Prostatic Hypertrophy.*

**Brachytherapy:** A form of radiation therapy in which radioactive seeds are implanted into the prostate to deliver radiation directly to the tumor. Also referred to as seed implantation, or seeding.

**Cancer:** A cellular malignancy typically forming tumors. Unlike benign tumors, these tend to invade surrounding tissues and spread to distant sites of the body.

**Carcinoma:** A malignant tumor made up chiefly of epithelial cells, or those cells that form the lining of an organ or cavity. *See Adenocarcinoma.*

**Castrate Range:** The level of the body's testosterone after orchiectomy (also referred to as castration). This is the range or level, which is used by physicians as a point of comparison for those drugs, which attempt to decrease the testosterone level.

**CAT Scan (or CT Scan):** *See Computer Tomography.*

**cGy:** Abbreviation for centigray; a unit of radiation equivalent to the older unit called a "rad."

**Chemotherapy:** The treatment of cancer using chemicals that deter the growth of cancer cells.

**Collimator:** A device that organizes radiation such that only parallel rays or beams emanate.

**Combination Hormonal Therapy (CHT):** Also referred to as Combined Hormonal Blockade (CHB), or Combined Androgen Deprivation Therapy (ADT). The preferred term is ADT, often designated with a number referring to the number of agents used (i.e., monotherapy ADT, ADT2, ADT3). This combined therapy can utilize a number of mechanisms, including surgical or medical ADT, antiandrogens, 5-alpha reductase inhibitors, estrogenic compounds, agents that block adrenal androgen production, and agents that decrease the receptivity of the androgen receptor.

**Combination Therapy:** Refers generally to any combination of treatment modalities used to treat prostate cancer.

**Computer Tomography:** Computer generated cross-sectional images of a portion of the body. Also called CT or CAT scan.

**Conformal Radiotherapy:** A radiation treatment conforming precisely to the size and shape of the prostate, with the use of computerized planning and state-of-the-art imaging techniques. 3-Dimensional Conformal Radiation Therapy (3D-CRT) utilizes this sophisticated approach to treatment planning, as does the even more advanced Intensity Modulated Radiation Therapy (IMRT).

**Cryosurgery (also referred to as Cryotherapy or Cryoablation):** The freezing of tissue with the use of liquid nitrogen or Argon gas probes. When used to treat prostate cancer, the cryoprobes are guided by transrectal ultrasound.

**Cytokine:** Any of a class of immunoregulatory substances that are secreted by cells of the immune system.

**DHT (dihydrotestosterone):** The active form of the male hormone, testosterone, produced after testosterone is transformed by an enzyme known as 5-alpha reductase.

**Diagnosis:** Evaluation of a patient's symptoms and/or test results, with the intent of identifying and verifying the existence of any underlying disease or abnormal condition.

**Digital Rectal Examination (DRE):** A procedure in which the physician inserts a gloved, lubricated finger into the rectum to examine the prostate gland for signs of cancer.

**DNA (Deoxyribonucleic Acid):** A complex protein that is the carrier of genetic information that determines the physical development and growth of living organisms.

**Doppler Ultrasound Technique:** A machine that sends out ultrasonic waves that pick up the velocity of blood flow through the veins and are transmitted as sound to make an image.

**Doubling Time:** The time it takes for a tumor or cancerous focus to double in size.

**Downsizing:** The use of hormonal therapy or other forms of intervention to reduce tumor volume prior to primary, curative treatment.

**Downstaging:** The use of hormonal therapy or other forms of intervention to lower the clinical stage of prostate cancer prior to primary, curative treatment.

**Ejaculatory Ducts:** The tubular passages through which semen reaches the prostatic urethra during orgasm.

**Ejaculation:** The release of semen through the penis during orgasm.

**Endorectal MRI:** Magnetic resonance imaging of the prostate gland using a probe inserted into the rectum. Dynamic Contrast Enhanced MRI is the most effective form of magnetic resonance imaging.

**Enzyme:** A chemical substance produced by living cells that causes chemical reactions to take place while not being changed itself.

**Erectile Dysfunction (also referred to as ED or impotence):** The loss of ability to produce and/or sustain an erection sufficient for intercourse.

**Estrogen:** A female sex hormone that can be used as a form of therapy to inhibit the production of testosterone in patients diagnosed with prostate cancer.

**External Beam Radiation Therapy (EBRT):** A form of radiation therapy that utilizes radiation delivered by an external source (machine) and directed at a target area to be radiated. In contrast to EBRT, brachytherapy utilizes radiation sources (seeds) that are internal, implanted in the target tissue. EBRT may use conventional photons, protons, neutrons or electrons.

**Extraprostatic Extension:** Used to describe prostate cancer that has spread outside the prostate gland.

**False Negative:** An erroneous negative test result. For example, an imaging test that fails to show the presence of a cancer tumor later found by biopsy to be present in the patient is said to have returned a false negative result.

**False Positive:** A positive test result that mistakenly identifies a state or condition that does not in fact exist.

**Feraheme (Ferumoxytol):** A ferromagnetic nanoparticle which is taken up by normal macrophages with the lymph nodes.

**Fistula:** With regard to prostate cancer, an abnormal passage due to injury or disease that connects an abscess or hollow organ to the surface of the body or to another hollow organ. If there is significant damage to the rectal wall proximate to the bladder, a fistula may occur between the bladder and rectum.

**Flare Reaction:** A testosterone surge caused by the initial use of an LHRH analog, causing a temporary increase of tumor growth and symptoms (known as clinical flare), or an increase in PSA (biochemical flare).

**Foley Catheter:** A catheter inserted in the penis and threaded through the urethra to the bladder where it is held in place with a tiny, inflated balloon. It removes urine from the bladder and can be used to irrigate the urethra and prevent blood clots.

**Free PSA:** PSA that is unattached to any major protein in the blood. Free PSA is associated with benign prostate growth. The percentage of free PSA is derived by dividing the free-PSA level by the total-PSA x 100. Studies have show that men with free PSA % > 25% were at low risk for prostate cancer, while men with PSA % < 10% were at high risk for having prostate cancer.

**Frozen Section:** A technique in which removed tissue is frozen, cut into thin slices, and stained for microscopic examination. A pathologist can rapidly

**complete a frozen section analysis, and for this reason, it is commonly used during surgery to quickly provide the surgeon with vital information.

**Gland:** An aggregation of cells (a structure or organ) that secretes a substance for use or discharge from the body.

**Gland Volume:** The size in cubic centimeters (cc) or grams of the prostate gland.

**Gleason Score:** A widely used method for classifying the cellular differentiation of cancerous tissue. The less the cancerous cells appear like normal cells, the more malignant the cancer. Two grades of 1-5, identifying the two most common degrees of differentiation present in the examined tissue sample, are added together to produce the Gleason score. High numbers indicate greater differentiation and more aggressive cancer. The grading system is named after its originator, Donald Gleason, M.D.

**Globulin:** Any of a number of simple proteins that occur widely in plant and animal tissues.

**Gynecomastia:** A side effect involving breast enlargement and tenderness, associated with various hormonal therapies that increase the level of estrogens in the body.

**HDR brachytherapy:** High Dose Rate brachytherapy involves the temporary insertion of radioactive iridium isotopes into the prostate gland using transrectal ultrasound guidance.

**Hematuria:** Blood in the urine.

**Hereditary:** Inherited genetically from parents and earlier generations.

**Holistic Medicine:** Medical care, which considers the patient as a whole, including his or her physical, mental, emotional, spiritual, social and economic needs.

**Hormone:** A substance produced by one tissue or gland and transported by the bloodstream to another to effect or regulate physiological activity such as metabolism and growth.

**Hormonal therapy:** Cancer treatment involving the blockage of hormone production by surgical or chemical means. Because prostate cancer is usually dependent on male hormones to grow, hormonal therapy can be an effective means of alleviating symptoms and retarding the development of the disease.

**Hormone refractory prostate cancer:** Prostate cancer that is androgen independent, and therefore, unresponsive to hormonal therapies.

**Hot Flash:** A side effect of some forms of hormonal therapy, experienced as a sudden rush of warmth to the face, neck, and upper body.

**Imaging:** Radiology techniques that are often computer-enhanced and allow the physician to visualize areas inside the body that would not normally be visible.

**Impotence:** *See Erectile Dysfunction.*

**Incontinence:** A loss of urinary control. There are various kinds and degrees of incontinence. Overflow incontinence is a condition in which the bladder retains urine after voiding. As a consequence, the bladder remains full most of the time, resulting in involuntary seepage of urine from the bladder. Stress incontinence is the involuntary discharge of urine when there is increased pressure upon the bladder, as in coughing or straining to lift heavy objects. Total incontinence is the failure of ability to voluntarily exercise control over the sphincters of the bladder neck and urethra, resulting in total loss of retentive ability.

**Inflammation:** Redness or swelling caused by injury or infection.

**Informed Consent:** Permission to proceed given by a patient after being fully informed of the purposes and potential consequences of a medical procedure.

**Intensity Modulated Radiation Therapy (IMRT):** The most recent state-of-the-art, computer-aided technique for delivering higher doses of radiation more accurately than either conventional External Beam Radiation or Conformal Radiation. The most advanced form of IMRT is Dynamic Adaptive Radiotherapy (DART).

**Intermittent Androgen Deprivation (IAD):** A temporary discontinuation of hormonal therapy that allows for a return to natural testosterone production in order to spare the patient from symptoms associated with androgen deprivation. Also referred to as Intermittent Hormonal Therapy (IHT).

**Intravenous Pyelogram (IVP):** A test that utilizes the injection of a special dye to check for injury or the spread of cancer to the kidneys and bladder.

**Investigational:** A drug or procedure allowed by the FDA for use in clinical trails, but not necessarily reimbursed.

**Isodose Line:** A line or two-dimensional shape that circumscribes an area receiving a radiation dose greater than or equal to a specified amount.

**Laparoscopic Lymphadenectomy:** The removal of pelvic lymph nodes with a laparoscope via four small incisions in the lower abdomen.

**LH (Luteinizing Hormone):** A chemical signal originating in the pituitary gland that causes the testes to make testosterone.

**LHRH Analogs (or LHRH Agonists):** Synthetic compounds that are chemically similar to Luteinizing Hormone Releasing Hormone (LHRH), used to suppress testicular production of testosterone. The most commonly prescribed LHRH analogs are Lupron® and Zoldex® Eligard® and Trelstar®. *See also Luteinizing Hormone-Releasing Hormone (LHRH).*

**LHRH Antagonist:** A chemical agent that blocks the LHRH receptor without the testosterone surge associated with LHRH analogs. LHRH antagonists include Abarelix (Plenaxis®).

**Linear Accelerator:** A high energy x-ray machine generating radiation fields for external beam radiation therapy. These machines are typically mounted with a collimator (or multileaf collimator) in a gantry that rotates vertically around the patient being treated.

**Localized Prostate Cancer:** Cancer that is confined to the prostate gland, and therefore, considered curable.

**Luteinizing Hormone-Releasing Hormone (LHRH):** A chemical signal originating in the hypothalamus that causes the pituitary to make LH, which in turn stimulates the testicles to make testosterone.

**Lymphadenectomy:** The removal and examination of lymph nodes to precisely diagnose and stage cancer. *See also Laparascopic Lymphadenectomy.*

**Lymph Node:** A small, bean-shaped mass of tissue located throughout the body along the vessels of the lymphatic system. The lymph nodes filter out bacteria and other toxins, as well as cancer cells.

**Magnetic Resonance Imaging (MRI):** A painless, non-invasive technique using strong magnetic fields to produce detailed images of internal body structures. An MRI scan usually takes about 45 minutes per site.

**Malignancy:** A tumorous growth of cancer cells.

**Malignant:** Having the invasive and metastatic properties of cancer. Tending to become progressively worse and to result in death.

**Margin:** *See Surgical Margin.*

**Metalloprotease Inhibitors:** Drugs used to suppress the body's production of certain enzymes.

**Metastasis:** The spread of cancer, by way of the blood stream or lymphatic system, beyond the boundaries of the organ or structure where the cancer originated. Metastases is the plural. Metastatic refers to the characteristics associated with cancer that has spread or a secondary tumor.

**Metastatic Work-Up:** A group of tests, including bone scans, x-rays, and blood tests, to ascertain whether cancer has metastasized.

**Monoclonal Antibody (mAb):** An antibody that is directed against one specific protein (antigen).

**Morbidity:** Unhealthy consequences and complications resulting from treatment.

**MRI:** *See Magnetic Resonance Imaging.*

**Nadir:** The lowest point. Doctors sometimes use this as a verb to describe return of cancer or treatment failure. The PSA nadir refers to a minimum PSA value that should be maintained after treatment if the cancer has been successfully eradicated.

**Necrosis:** Death of cells or tissues caused by disease or injury.

**Neoadjuvant:** The use of a different type of therapy before primary, curative treatment. For example, neoadjuvant Androgen Deprivation Therapy is often used prior to radiation therapy or radical surgery, with the intent of improving the effectiveness of the primary treatment by reducing the size of the tumor and/or prostate gland.

**Nerve-sparing:** A procedure used during radical prostatectomy in which the surgeon attempts to save the nerves (neurovascular bundles) that allow for normal sexual functions.

**Neurovascular Bundles:** Strands of interwoven nerves and veins that run down the side of the prostate. The bundles contain microscopic nerves that are essential for erection; they also contain arteries and veins. Cutting the nerves in the bundles during surgery, or otherwise harming them in another procedure, usually renders the patient impotent.

**Nocturia:** Getting up at night to urinate.

**Non-invasive:** Not involving any incision in the body.

**Oncogenes:** Genes associated with tumor growth.

**Oncology:** The branch of medical science dealing with tumors. A medical oncologist is a specialist in the study of cancerous tumors.

**Organ-confined Disease (OCD):** Prostate cancer that is confined to the prostate gland, as indicated clinically or pathologically.

**Orchiectomy:** A simple operation that involves surgical removal of the testicles, which produce most of the body's testosterone.

**Osteoporosis:** A decrease in bone mass and density causing fragility and porosity.

**Overstaging:** An assessment of an overly high clinical stage at initial diagnosis.

**Palliative:** Affording symptomatic pain relieve but not cure or remission.

**Palpable:** Capable of being felt when examined by touch or manipulation.

**PAP:** *See Prostatic Acid Phosphatase.*

**Pathologist:** A doctor who specializes in the examination of cells and tissues removed from the body.

**PBRT:**
*See Proton Beam Radiation Therapy.*

**Perineum:** The area of the body between the anus and scrotum. A perineal procedure uses this area as the point of entry into the body.

**Perineural Invasion:** Describing cancer, which has spread from the prostate to the nerve bundles.

**Periprostatic:** Relating to the soft tissues immediately proximate to the prostate gland.

**Photon:** The quantum of electromagnetic energy, described as having zero mass and no electric charge. X-rays are high energy photons.

**Placebo:** A sugar pill often taken by participants in a medical study. Patients taking a placebo are compared to patients taking actual medications.

**Ploidy Analysis:** A pathological analysis to determine the number of sets of chromosomes in a cell.

**Proctitis:** Inflammation of the rectum.

**Prognosis:** A forecast of the course of a disease and future prospects of the patient.

**Progression:** A change in the status of the cancer indicating the condition has progressed and worsened.

**Pro-oxidant:** A term to describe substances that aid in oxidation.

**ProstaScint® Scan:** An imaging technique sometimes used determine whether or not cancer has spread to distant sites by using monoclonal antibodies.

**Prostate Capsule:** It was once thought that the prostate gland was surrounded by a clearly identifiable capsule, but pathological studies have shown there is no capsule as such. The gland exists within a fat plane.

**Prostatectomy:** The surgical removal of part or all of the prostate gland.

**Prostate Specific Antigen (PSA):** A blood test that measures a substance manufactured solely by prostate gland cells. An elevated reading indicates an abnormal condition of the prostate gland, either benign or malignant. It is presently the most sensitive tumor marker for the identification and monitoring of prostate cancer.

**Prostatic Acid Phosphatase (PAP):** An enzyme produced by the prostate that is elevated (3.0 or higher) in many patients when prostate cancer has spread beyond the prostate.

**Prostatitis:** An infection or inflammation of the prostate gland that is treatable with medications.

**Proton Beam Radiation Therapy (PBRT):** A form of radiation therapy that utilizes protons as the source of energy (as opposed to X-rays or neutrons).

**PSA:** *See Prostate Specific Antigen.*

**PSA Bounce (or PSA Bump):** A rise in PSA level after first having a reduction in PSA after radiation therapy.

**PSA Nadir:** The lowest PSA value after a particular treatment.

**PSA Velocity (PSAV):** The rate of increase of the PSA level, expressed as nanograms per milliliter per year.

**Radiation Therapy (RT):** The use of high energy rays to kill cancer cells and malignant tissue.

**Radiation Urethritis:** Inflammation of the urethra caused by radiation therapy.

**Radical Prostatectomy:** An operation to remove the entire prostate gland and seminal vesicles.

**Radiosensitivity:** The degree to which a type of cancer responds to radiation therapy.

**RBA or Relative Biological Effectiveness:** A scale used to compare the intensity of radiation associated with various atomic particles.

**Receptor:** A cellular docking site that interacts with a specific protein or enzyme (called a ligand). The interaction typically leads to the synthesis of other substances such as proteins, hormones or enzymes.

**Recurrence:** Return of the cancer following remission or treatment intended as curative. Local recurrence indicates a return of the cancer at the site of origin. Distant recurrence indicates the appearance of one or more metastases of the disease.

**Refractory:** A term indicating that the cancer no longer responds to the current therapy.

**Remission:** Complete or partial disappearance of the signs and symptoms of the disease. The period during which a disease remains under control, without progressing. Even complete remission does not necessarily indicate cure.

**Resection:** The surgical removal of a part of an organ or structure.

**Risk:** The probability that a particular event will or will not happen.

**RP:** *See Radical Prostatectomy.*

**RT:** *See Radiation Therapy.*

**Rx:** The standard abbreviation for prescription.

**Salvage Treatment:** A medical term for "Plan B." It means a patient must undergo another form of treatment because the first therapy was not successful. Salvage therapy may incur a higher rate of side effects.

**Saw Palmetto:** A nutrient extracted from the saw palmetto shrub, which is considered by some to aid the body's immune system.

**Seed Implantation (SI):** A minimally invasive procedure by which radioactive seeds are implanted into the prostate gland to destroy cancer. Also referred to as seeding and brachytherapy.

**Selenium:** A non-metallic element thought to be beneficial as a nutrient; it is often included in multivitamin supplements.

**Seminal Vesicles:** Glands that, like the prostate, support male reproduction. Fluid secreted by these glands regulates the consistency of semen.

**Side Effect:** A reaction to a treatment or medication, usually referring to an undesirable effect.

**Sphincter:** A circular muscle which contracts to close an orifice. The urethral sphincter squeezes the urethra shut, providing urinary control.

**Staging:** The testing process by which the extent and severity of a known cancer is evaluated according to an established system of classification. It is used to help determine appropriate therapy. *See TNM Staging and Whitmore-Jewett Staging.*

**Surgical Margin:** The outer edge of the tissue removed during a radical prostatectomy. The surgical margin may be "negative," indicating that no cancer is present and a better prognosis, or "positive," indicating that not all of the cancer has been removed.

**Systemic:** Throughout the body and affecting the entire body.

**T-Cell:** An immune system cell or lymphocyte that directs an immune response to malignant or infected cells.

**Testes:** Two male reproductive glands located inside the scrotum. The testes are the primary sources for testosterone. Also called testicles.

**Testosterone:** A male sex hormone chiefly produced by the testicles.

**Thrombotic:** Causing or relating to blood clotting.

**TNM Staging:** The most widely used classification system for evaluating the extent of prostate cancer. TNM refers to tumor, nodes and metastases. *See Staging.*

**Transrectal:** Through the rectum.

**Transurethral:** Through the urethra.

**Transrectal Ultrasonography:** *See Ultrasound.*

**Transurethral Resection of the Prostate (TURP):** A surgical procedure to remove tissue obstructing the urethra. The technique involves the insertion of an instrument called a resectoscope into the penile urethra, and is intended to relieve obstruction of urine flow due to enlargement of the prostate.

**Tumor:** An excessive growth of cells that is caused by uncontrolled and disorderly cell replacement. Abnormal tissue growth may be benign or malignant. See also Benign, Malignant.

**TURP:** *See Transurethral Resection of the Prostate.*

**Ultrasound (Transrectal Ultrasonography):** A painless, non-invasive diagnostic imaging technique using sound waves to create an echo pattern that reveals the structure of organs and tissues. It does not use x-rays.

**Understaging:** An overly low assessment of clinical stage at diagnosis.

**Urethra:** The tube that carries urine from the bladder and semen from the prostate out of the body through the penis.

**Urologist:** A physician who specializes in the diagnosis and the medical and surgical treatment of problems in the urinary and male reproductive systems.

**USPIO:** This technology uses ultra-small superparamagnetic iron oxide (USPIO) as an MRI contrast agent for the identification of cancer metastasis in lymph nodes.

**Vasectomy:** A surgical procedure to render a man sterile by cutting the vas deferens, thus eliminating the passage of sperm from the testes to the prostate.

**Vasoactive:** Causing the dilation or constriction of blood vessels.

**Vesicle:** A small sac containing fluid, as in seminal vesicles.

**Whitmore-Jewett Staging:** A classification system for evaluating the extent of prostate cancer. This system is less widely used for the designation of stage than is TNM staging.

**X-rays:** High energy radiation that can be used at low levels of intensity to make images of the body's internal structures, or at high intensity for radiation therapy.

# ABOUT THE AUTHOR

## Michael J. Dattoli, MD

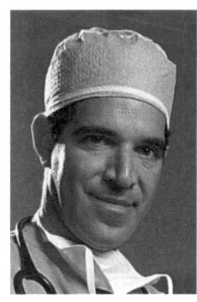

Michael J. Dattoli, MD, is a board-certified radiation oncologist with well over two decades of brachytherapy experience and has performed thousands of prostate implant procedures. He is considered the foremost pioneer in the field, optimizing brachytherapy designs to maximize tumor eradication and minimize symptoms. He has also been the leading trailblazer in the development of Dynamic Adaptive Radiotherapy (DART), utilizing all of the state-of-the-art modalities associated with 4-Dimensional Image-Guided Intensity Modulated Radiotherapy (3D-IMRT). Dr. Dattoli has successfully applied the same technologies to other forms of cancer, including breast, head and neck, GI, GYN, sarcomas and lung malignancies. He is a noted author and speaker in this complex field of medicine.

Dr. Dattoli attended the University of California at Berkeley and was the Valedictorian of his class at Vassar College; he earned his medical degree at Mount Sinai School of Medicine, Radiation Oncology at New York University Medical Center, then distinguished himself at Memorial Sloan-Kettering Cancer Center and New York Hospital-Cornell University Medical Center, as the Special Fellow in Brachytherapy. He was appointed Associate Professor in Brachytherapy and Radiation Oncology at Memorial Sloan- Kettering Cancer Center in New York and at New York Hospital-Cornell University Medical Center prior to relocating to Florida.

Dr. Dattoli also serves on multiple journal editorial review boards. Government appointments include "The Prostate Cancer Task Force" in Florida and consultant to the "Washington Oncology Roundtable Advisory Committee". He was selected by the International Association of Oncologists as a Leading Physician of the World and top Brachytherapist.

# THE DATTOLI CANCER FOUNDATION MISSION

The Dattoli Cancer Foundation, sponsor of the Prostate Cancer Resource Network, is a 501(c)(3), tax-exempt charitable organization, whose mission is

- to raise awareness of the wide-spread incidence of Prostate Cancer and the need for early and annual screenings;

- to provide information and support to men newly diagnosed with Prostate Cancer as well as to those with recurrent Prostate Cancer, and

- to foster research into better diagnostic tools and treatment options for Prostate Cancer.

*Gifts to the Dattoli Foundation make possible publications like this one, and are welcomed anytime. A copy of the official registration and financial information may be obtained from the Division of Consumer Services by calling toll-free (800-435-7352) within the state. Registration does not imply endorsement, approval or recommendations by the state.*

**Dattoli Cancer Foundation**
2803 Fruitville Road
Sarasota, FL 34237
941/365-5599
800/915-1001
fax: 941/330-2317
www.dattolifoundation.org

# ORDER MORE BOOKLETS IN THE SERIES

This *Prostate Cancer Essentials for Survival* booklet was published by the Dattoli Cancer Foundation. For a complete list of booklets in the series and ordering information, please visit the Dattoli Cancer Center Book Shelf at dattoli.com/book-shelf. Current titles include::

- ✔ *Conquering Prostate Cancer with DART and Brachytherapy*
- ✔ *The Dattoli Prostate Cancer Challenge: Evaluating All Your Treatment Options*
- ✔ *The Facts: Comparing Prostate Cancer Treatment Options*
- ✔ *Interpreting Your PSA Results and Related Prostate Cancer Lab Tests*
- ✔ *Dynamic Adaptive Radiotherapy*
- ✔ *Image-Guided Prostate Biopsy: When, Why and What to Expect*
- ✔ *Dosimetry and Prostate Cancer Radiotherapy*
- ✔ *Advanced Imaging for Prostate Cancer: A Primer on 3D Color-Flow Power Doppler Ultrasound, Multiparametric MRI and CT Fusion Techniques*
- ✔ *Radiation Safety and Prostate Cancer: Need You Be Concerned?*
- ✔ *Hormonal Therapy for Prostate Cancer: The Benefits and Risks*
- ✔ *The Dattoli Blue Ribbon Prostate Cancer Solution: How to Survive and Thrive Without Surgery*

# THE WARNING SIGNS OF PROSTATE CANCER

There are often no warning signs of prostate cancer. In some cases the following symptoms may indicate the presence of the disease. However, please be aware that these symptoms may also be due to benign conditions of the prostate, or other conditions entirely unrelated to prostate cancer:

- ✔ Elevated or rising PSA
- ✔ Abnormal Digital Rectal Exam
- ✔ Blood in urine
- ✔ Pain or difficulty urinating
- ✔ Increased urge to urinate, especially at night
- ✔ Hesitant or intermittent urinary flow
- ✔ Pain or discomfort in area of prostate
- ✔ Unusual and unexplained weight loss
- ✔ Continual pain in lower back, hips or pelvis
- ✔ Increased voiding urgency
- ✔ Inability to urinate
- ✔ Trouble having or keeping an erection (erectile dysfunction)
- ✔ Weakness or numbness in the legs or feet

www.ingramcontent.com/pod-product-compliance
Lightning Source LLC
Chambersburg PA
CBHW040226220526
45473CB00001B/144